THE INDISPENSABLE
GUIDE TO PANCREAS

SHANNON ADAMS

Dedication

This book is dedicated to my father, a decorated Vietnam War veteran and Chaplain, who passed away from pancreatic cancer in August of 2015.

This book is also dedicated to other pancreatic cancer patients and their loved ones so that their journey with this disease might be a bit easier than it was for my dad and me.

Copyright © 2016 Shannon Adams All Rights Reserved

TABLE OF CONTENTS

CHAPTER ONE: OUR STORY

CHAPTER TWO: WHAT IS PANCREATIC CANCER

CHAPTER THREE: SYMPTOMS OF PANCREATIC CANCER

CHAPTER FOUR: TESTING FOR PANCREATIC CANCER

CHAPTER FIVE: STATISTICS AND STAGING FOR PANCREATIC CANCER

CHAPTER SIX: GAME PLAN FOR PANCREATIC CANCER

CHAPTER SEVEN: QUESTIONS FOR PRIMARY DOCTOR AND/OR ONCOLOGIST

CHAPTER EIGHT: UNDERSTANDING THE NUANCES OF PANCREATIC CANCER

CHAPTER NINE: PERFORMANCE STATUS

CHAPTER TEN: PANCREATIC CANCER TREATMENT OPTIONS

CHAPTER ELEVEN: RESEARCH INTO PANCREATIC CANCER TREATMETNS

CHAPTER TWELVE: SYMPTOMS OF PANCREATIC CANCER AND SIDE EFFECTS OF CANCER TREATMENTS

CHAPTER THIRTEEN: SURGICAL PROCEDURES THAT MAY BE NEEDED FOR THOSE WITH PANCREATIC CANCER

CHAPTER FOURTEEN: SCREENINGS AND ONGOING SCREENINGS

CHAPTER FIFTEEN: WHEN SHOULD AN ER VISIT BE MADE

CHAPTER SIXTEEN: SUPPORT

CHAPTER SEVENTEEN: HOSPICE AND THE DYING PROCESS

CHAPTER EIGHTEEN: LEGAL DOCUMENTS

CHAPTER ONE

OUR STORY

Jaundice

At the beginning of July 2015, my 85 year old father went to the doctor for a routine checkup and blood work. When he returned for his test results his doctor told him that his liver enzymes were elevated. His doctor became alarmed because my father's skin had a yellowish hue to it. When someone's skin turns yellow, the medical community terms this as being "jaundiced". Being jaundiced in and of itself is not deadly. Jaundice is a symptom of several different underlying medical conditions that can cause death if left untreated. Normally, jaundice is caused by a gallstone that is blocking the bile duct. A typical gallstone that gets stuck in the bile duct can easily be removed with surgery.

Quick Lesson on the Gallbladder, Pancreas and Bile Duct

Bile is a liquid substance that our livers produce daily to help our body digest fats that we eat. It is a greenish color. Each day, about 27-34 ounces of bile travels from the liver into the **gallbladder** (which stores some bile). After we eat, the gallbladder will send an appropriate amount of bile down the **bile duct** (a tube) into the small intestines. When the bile is just about to enter into the small intestines, it passes by a **pancreatic duct** which squeezes some pancreatic juices in with the bile. After the pancreatic juices and bile enter the small intestines – they work together to digest the food we consume.

Jaundice changes the colors of the skin, urine and stool. If anything causes a blockage along the bile duct, then the bile cannot exit the body and backs up into our blood stream. People get a **yellow hue to their skin**, eyes and organs as the bile enters the bloodstream. The bile is then filtered by the kidneys which, in turn causes the **urine to become a dark tea color**. Since bile gives human stool the normal brown color, human **stool will become a very pale clay color**. Once the bile duct blockage is corrected, then the stool will return to a normal brown color and the urine will return to a normal pale yellow color.

If the bile duct remains blocked for an extended period of time, eventually the liver will become diseased and fail. In addition, as bile builds up, the gallbladder may rupture. Humans cannot survive unless the liver functions properly; therefore, bile duct blockages must be medically treated as soon as possible.

The First ER Visit

After finding that my father had jaundice, the doctor insisted that he go to the local Emergency Room right away. Physically, my dad did felt fine and was not in pain, but he went home and prepared for a hospital stay. His close friend picked him up and brought him to the Emergency Room.

I lived out of state and spoke to my dad a few times a day to find out what was happening. He complained that not much was being done since it was the weekend, but he took comfort in knowing that the reason they probably admitted him on Friday was to ensure that he would be one of the first to be taken care of Monday morning. Unfortunately, the hospital television didn't carry the Yankees' games.

At the hospital, the doctors ordered tests. An ultrasound and a CT scan indicated that indeed, something was blocking his bile duct. Also, his gallbladder had many gallstones in it. It was presumed that a gallstone was blocking the bile duct and needed removal to relieve the jaundice.

On Monday morning, a surgical gastroenterologist performed what is called an ERCP. My dad was put under anesthesia. A tube was snaked down his throat, through his stomach, into the small intestines (duodenum) and up through the small bile duct tube that normally drains bile into the small intestines. The surgeon tried to remove the stone, but could only get a couple of pieces of the stone to break free. The surgeon felt the stone was impacted and aborted the remainder of the procedure. When my dad woke up, the surgeon told my dad that they were sending him to another hospital the next day to have a specialist surgeon remove the impacted gallstone.

Since my parents' divorce 10 years earlier, my father had lived on his own. It was customary for my dad to call me whenever he was being discharged from a hospital so that I could help care for him during his recovery. This time was different. On Monday night, after his first procedure, he asked me to come right away. As far as I knew, his only problem was that he had a gallstone blocking his bile duct, but I could sense fear in his voice. He needed me to be there. The next day, I arrived by plane.

On Tuesday, my dad was transported to see the expert gastrointestinal surgeon to have another ERCP to remove the gallstone. They didn't return him to the local hospital until early Wednesday morning, so I camped out at his house until Wednesday morning when visiting hours started at 9:00 am.

Probable Pancreatic Cancer

On Wednesday morning before visiting hours, my dad called me from the hospital and told me that the doctor diagnosed him with pancreatic cancer. I was shocked and so was he. I drove straight to the hospital. The visiting center people were reluctant to let me up before visiting hours, but I told them that my father had just been diagnosed with cancer and that I was to meet with him and his doctors right away. They agreed to let me go up.

I went to his room and my dad was lying comfortably in his hospital bed. He appeared concerned and I told him I didn't understand how they could have diagnosed him with pancreatic cancer when the ERCP procedure didn't even take place in his pancreas. We were both perplexed. I told him that I would talk to his doctor.

I asked the nurse for the name and phone number of the doctor who had given my dad that horrible news and I left a message with the doctor's office.

The doctor returned my call at noon and told me that he had not diagnosed my dad "officially" with pancreatic cancer, but that it most likely was pancreatic cancer. During the second ERCP procedure, the surgeon saw that both the bile duct and pancreatic duct were **strictured (narrowed)**. The surgeon had inserted a stent (tube) to open up the bile duct to relieve the jaundice. The surgeon felt that the reason that both of the ducts were narrowed was due to a tumor growing in the head of my father's pancreas which was pressing the bile duct closed.

I left the hospital to let my dad rest and planned to return later. My dad's friends had asked me to join them at their weekly early bird dinner at 4:00 pm. I agreed to join them with the intention of seeing my dad afterwards.

Going Home After First Hospitalization

At about 3:30 pm, my father called me and said he was being discharged! I cancelled my early bird dinner plans and went to get him. After the hospital tech helped him into the car, he insisted that we stop by the restaurant on the way home. He hated missing his daily outings with his buddies. I reluctantly agreed to bring him to the restaurant.

I did not know a single thing about pancreatic cancer, and had been researching the disease all afternoon. I had already discovered, through my research, that pancreatic cancer tended to be a quick killer with the average person having only 3-6 months of life left after diagnosis. Knowing someone you love has cancer quickly changes one's mindset. It wasn't about him "being careful" anymore - now, it was about him enjoying what time he had left. We were off to see his friends at the restaurant.

With a cane in one hand and me holding his other arm for stability, my dad wobbled into the restaurant and sat down at a table filled with his friends. His buddies were so glad to see him and they immediately ripped the hospital band off of his arm. He had a sip of his favorite drink, Jameson's Irish Whiskey, along with a bit of potato skin. After 30 minutes, he was ready to go home, rest and recuperate. It was now my turn to take care of him which entailed fixing meals, cleaning, laundry and making sure he could get around safely.
He was extremely tired from having the 2 ERCP procedures done. His jaundice was clearing up quite nicely and his skin was returning to a normal color.

This trip was different from the others I had previously taken. Once home, my dad suffered from 2.5 days of severe diarrhea. We thought it might be because he switched to a new medication. During his diarrhea bouts, I had to go get him some smaller anti-diarrheal pills because he was having difficulty swallowing the regular sized anti-diarrheal medication. I got him the smaller pills, but it concerned me because the regular pills were so tiny to begin with. I had never known him to have much trouble swallowing. In addition, I found that I needed to cut his food up into tiny pieces for him to be able to eat it. And finally, my dad always was up early and I had never seen him sleep in before, but during this trip he slept in until about 9:00 am daily.

Later that night, I spent hours researching pancreatic cancer, strictured bile ducts and strictured pancreatic ducts. I found that if both the bile duct and pancreatic ducts are narrowed that this is referred to as a **"Double Duct Sign"**. Having the Double Duct Sign is highly indicative of pancreatic cancer. The bile duct and pancreatic duct travel through the head of the pancreas. If a cancerous tumor grows in the head of the pancreas, it can put pressure on both the bile duct and pancreatic duct – causing them both to narrow. As the tumor grows, the narrowing can get worse until both ducts are completely pinched off.

Six Month Stock-Up and the Waiting Game

On Thursday, after preparing his breakfast and ensuring he was relaxed and snug in his special recliner, I went to the grocery store and stocked up on a 6 month supply of Cheerios, canned peaches, green tea, frozen raspberries, toilet paper and 6 months of other necessities he would need. Walking up and down the supermarket isles, trying to remember his favorites, I was overcome with sadness in that I was doing some of his final shopping for him. During his final 3-6 months, the last thing he needed to worry about was groceries, so I tried to do as much as possible for him before I had to go back home again.

On Thursday night, as he watched the Yankees game in his favorite reclining chair - I fervently researched everything I could about pancreatic cancer. As an elderly man, he had little use for modern technology and accordingly, he had no internet access so I was relegated to using my smartphone. I was planning on going home on Sunday as I had many things to catch up on, but his doctor told him the biopsy results would not be back until the following Wednesday. My dad asked me to stay so I could go to the appointment with him. Of course, I agreed to stay as I knew he was frightened.

From Friday through Wednesday, we waited for the appointment that had been scheduled with his general practitioner. He was to receive his biopsy results. Although we had already been told it probably was pancreatic cancer - we hoped the biopsy would be negative. Unfortunately, my research found that even a negative biopsy did not indicate that he was cancer free. The surgeon had only performed a brush biopsy inside of his bile duct and had not retrieved a sample directly from the tumor in the pancreas. There was still hope though.

On Friday, I had purchased a book about pancreatic cancer and told my dad that the book was available if he wanted to be prepared with questions for the doctor. I told him I wouldn't bother him about it again, but it was there if he wanted to read it. He never asked to read it.

Throughout the week, dad's strength increased. He still wasn't eating very much, but his appetite was improving. His skin color was almost normal and he told me his urine was getting back to a "closer to normal" color. It was such a relief just to see his jaundice disappearing.

Dad had been a Chaplain in the military and served tours in the Vietnam War. Prior to the war, he had been ordained a Catholic Priest. He was a very religious man who had married after the Vietnam War. He had become my step-father when I was 3 years old and I am very appreciative of that. On Sunday, because he could not attend mass at the church down the street, he said mass for both of us in the dining room.

On Tuesday, outside of dad's earshot, I called the doctor's office. I asked if the biopsy results were in and she said that they were. At this point in time, I had typed up and printed 16 pages of research into pancreatic cancer. Dad didn't know it, but I was preparing for war against this cancer. I kept my research under wraps as I didn't want to worry or alarm him. His job for now was to regain his strength so that we could fight this thing.

Biopsy Results

On Wednesday, my dad told me that if the biopsy results were positive that he wanted to talk some things over. He didn't know that I was well aware of the prognosis, treatment options, where he could get treated and the transportation available to and from treatment. There was no way I could stay with him for 6 months or longer, so I looked up all sorts of social services to help him.

Nervous, we went to the appointment and the doctor looked dad over. He said the slight yellow tinge to dad's skin would take 2-3 weeks to completely clear. We asked him about the biopsy and he said the results had not come in yet. We were both disappointed as it had been an entire week since the biopsy had been taken and the girl in his office had said the day before that the biopsy results were in. I did not push the issue because I did not want to stress my dad out.

The doctor ordered a blood test to discover if dad's liver enzymes were lowering. I asked the doctor to also test his CA19-9 and the doctor said it wasn't necessary since we didn't have the biopsy results back yet. **CA19-9 is a pancreatic cancer tumor marker (a protein)** that can be found in higher levels in the blood of SOME pancreatic cancer patients. If the CA19-9 results were elevated, then it would have been a good indicator that dad had pancreatic cancer. I was disappointed that the doctor refused to do this test since it would have helped us plan for treatments regardless of the biopsy results.

At this point in time, my father was too weak to fight doctors over slow biopsy results and blood tests. My father looked to me to help him in this journey; however, I could not be a good advocate for my father because I lacked the knowledge about pancreatic cancer, bile ducts and brush biopsies. At the time, I did not "get" that waiting for the results of a bile duct brush biopsy was silly because the biopsy was from the inside of the bile duct and not directly from the tumor itself. **This meant that the biopsy would only have been positive if the tumor had actually invaded the bile duct. My father easily could have had pancreatic cancer regardless of whether the brush biopsy of the bile duct came back negative or not.**

The doctor proceeded to tell us that he could tell by examination that dad was a very sick man. Dejected, we went to get his blood test. In the waiting room, my dad worked up a conversation with another elderly man who had a cane with him as well. They both got called to take their blood tests simultaneously and my dad said, "I'll race you!"

After we returned home, I prepared a snack for my dad. I asked him what he wanted to do if the biopsy came back positive. He said that he would do chemo and radiation. By that time, I was suspicious that the doctor did not think treatment was an option for my father and that's why he was in no rush to obtain the biopsy results or test CA19-9 levels. My research later that night confirmed my suspicions. It seemed apparent that due to my dad's frail health (**Performance Status**), he would not qualify for any treatment. Of course, I didn't let on about my suspicions. I was no doctor and I didn't want to worry or scare my father who had hope.

On Wednesday night, the night before I left to fly back home, my dad asked me if I had watched the movie "Unbroken". I had already watched it, but it was a good movie and I didn't want my dad to fuss about me having already watched it - so I denied ever seeing it when he asked. We stayed up really late that night watching it. It was the story of an American Olympic Champion who was taken prisoner and relentlessly tortured by the Japanese during WWII. I did not know it at the time, but that movie would later help me to stay strong throughout my father's illness and death.

Thursday morning arrived and it was time for me to return home. My father had regained much of his strength, could drive his car again and was able to hang out with his buddies. I called often to check up on him. He sounded like he was feeling so much better.

The Second Hospitalization

A week and a day later, on a Friday afternoon, I received a phone call from my dad's neighbor. The neighbor told me that my dad was having a heart attack and they were waiting for an ambulance. I freaked out! My dad said he wanted me to come back up to New Jersey. Over the next 3 hours I wrapped up my work, bought a plane ticket and was ready to go out the door to the airport when my dad's friends told me not to come - that my father was feeling a lot better. The severe chest pain was gone. I reluctantly cancelled my plane ticket. The doctor said had he had not had a heart attack, but it was probably a cardiac related event.

That evening, unbeknownst to me, my dad was up most of the night vomiting and in pain. By Saturday, he felt better and the doctor discharged him. Upon discharge, and almost THREE WEEKS after the biopsy had been taken, the doctor finally told my dad that the brush biopsy was positive and that he did have pancreatic cancer.

My dad was really weak from being up all night vomiting and his buddy picked him up from the emergency room and brought him home. No one expected him to be discharged so soon. I was planning to fly up on Sunday but was unable to fly due to a system wide computer issue with the airlines. I would drove all day Sunday to get to him.

On Sunday, as I was driving, my dad slumped down on the bathroom floor due to weakness and couldn't get up. His buddies got his younger neighbor to come over and help him up. He was always so scared of falling and I wasn't there to help! I felt horrible. He decided to stay in bed until I could get to him on Monday.

MONDAY

On Monday, I opened the front door and my dad was standing in the kitchen with his cane. He was staring in a daze at his steeping green tea and his breakfast muffin. He was slow to say hello but was extremely relieved I was there. He told me he had just gotten up. I asked him to go sit down at the table so that I could bring his food to him.

He ate just a little bit and started to close his eyes and nod off. Not wanting him to fall out of his chair, I insisted he go back to sleep. It worried me to see him so weak. In helping him, I also noticed that his handheld urinal had dark urine in it. He got up Monday evening and was very weak. He requested cut up kielbasa sausage with scrambled eggs. I made his dinner as he requested and he only ate a handful, but he absolutely loved it and thanked me profusely.

TUESDAY

Tuesday morning, my dad slept in. I went to the home improvement store and got some mulch to spread throughout his flower beds. After he got up at 10 am, I made him breakfast and he said the bowl of cereal was too big to eat. I told him to eat what he could and he ate about a handful of Cheerios. I helped him get to his recliner so that he could relax.

It was so hard to see him struggle to stand, walk and sit. During these two days, for the first time ever, I had to help him remove and put on his shoes and shocks. He was using his cane and grabbing onto everything he could to keep himself stable. I thought it was strange that he was so weak considering he had not had a heart attack nor any procedures at the hospital. I figured that recent his bile duct hospitalization along with his recent "cardiac event" was what was making him weak.

His goal for Tuesday was to take a shower so that he could see his cardiologist the next morning. I told him that he was so weak that he would need a nap before he showered. He took a long nap and got up. He insisted that I stand just outside of the bathroom door while he showered in case he needed help (he was terrified of falling again). He was able to shower and he then settled into his recliner to watch television. That night, he requested the kielbasa and scrambled eggs again and I gladly obliged. He ate quite a bit of it with a piece of toast and I was happy to see him getting his appetite back.

Third Hospitalization

WEDNESDAY

Wednesday morning at 5:15 am, my dad called out my name. I ran into his room and he was vomiting. He told me he had been up all night vomiting and was nauseous. I asked him why he had not called out for me earlier and he said he had wanted me to get some rest! I renewed his small garbage can that had been soiled and put a wet washcloth on his head. He felt like he was a burning up. He started vomiting again. He didn't own a thermometer and his temperature concerned me. I ran out to the store to quickly purchase a thermometer. After I took his temperature, the thermometer read 103.5! I made him take it twice and it was the same. I went into the kitchen and took my temp and it was normal.

I told him that he had a very high fever and that he had to go back to the emergency room. He was agreeable. The ambulance came and the paramedics entered the front door that I had left open for them. They came into my dad's bedroom and tried to get my dad to get to stand up. He couldn't. It took 2 men to help him stand so that he could get into the ambulance chair-bed. I gathered his stuff and drove the 7 minutes it took to get to the hospital. I texted the update on my father's condition to one of his buddies.

In the emergency room, the person I had texted was already there. My father was in decent spirits, but told me his stomach hurt. I asked how bad the pain was and he told me a 10 out of 10! He said it had been hurting all night. I ran and got the nurse, told her that my father had pancreatic cancer and that his stomach was in terrible pain. She quickly got an order of morphine from the doctor. That morning, out of frustration, I told anyone who came into my dad's room that he needed a **Pancreatic Protocol CT Scan**. We needed to see what was going on! He started to get yellow again in the emergency room!

The doctor finally came in and diagnosed my father with **acute pancreatitis** (an inflammation of the pancreas). His pancreatic duct was strictured (narrowed) or blocked due to the pancreatic cancer tumor. After he ate dinner the prior night, his pancreas tried to send digestive juices through the pancreatic duct into the bile duct. Since there was a blockage, the pancreatic juices backed up into his pancreas and started to digest the pancreas itself. This caused a severe inflammation of the pancreas, the pain, vomiting and spiked fever.

My dad rested and I went back to the house to do some things for him. I notified my siblings and my brother wanted to fly out. I made plans to pick him up at the airport at 1:30 am that evening. I felt that this was another hospital episode which would require a maybe 4 days of dad being in the hospital and another 7-10 days of recuperation. I was hoping my brother could "take over" for me so that I could tend to some things at my home and then come right back to help. I left my dad about 5:00 pm to get to the airport in time to pick up my brother.

THURSDAY

Thursday morning, I was getting ready to visit dad. I planned on waking my brother up shortly and I was excited that my dad was going to be able to see my brother. It would be a nice treat to have both of us there to help him.

As I was getting ready, my dad's house phone began phone to ring and the caller ID voice prompter shouted out "Call from Hospital... Call from Hospital... Call from Hospital". I thought dad had died! I ran to answer it and it was one of my dad's doctors. He told me that the bile duct stent had failed and there wasn't anything they could do for him. He told me to ask for him when I got to the hospital.

I was worried sick. What did that mean!? Why couldn't they do anything!? They fixed the jaundice last time! I knew that there were medical options available to help my dad. They could remove his gallbladder, give him antibiotics and clear the stent blockage.

I immediately woke my brother up and we went straight to the hospital. When someone tells you that there's nothing more they can do, your heart aches for the person you love. You can't imagine that this is the end.

When we entered the hospital room, my dad said hello to me and my fiancé. I had to explain that the other man with me was not fiancé - it was my brother. Dad then recognized my brother and said hello with a big smile. My dad looked at me in a confused state and asked me where he was. I asked him where he thought he was. He paused and thought for a moment. He said that he was in the hospital and I said he was right. I thought maybe the morphine was causing him some confusion. I later learned that I should have just told him where he was instead of making him guess.

He was so happy to see my brother. We all talked for a whlle and then my dad complained about being in pain. I told him I would get a nurse to give him more morphine right away. He looked at me and said, "Morphine, yes…just like they used to give the guys." I responded, "Yes dad, just like they used to give the guys in Nam." My dad was a Chaplain during the Vietnam War and he was remembering all of the soldiers who were given morphine when they were dying. This was the first hint from my dad that he realized the end of his life was coming.

I immediately went to the nurses' station to request more morphine and to ask for the doctor who had called me earlier. The doctor came to the room pretty quickly.

The doctor told us that my dad's stent had failed and that probably a gallstone, an infection or another stricture along the bile duct was blocking the bile duct. He told my dad that he had a choice, he could have surgery to bypass the bile duct and have a bag outside of his body to collect the bile or he could go home on hospice. My dad was very weak, but he understood what the doctor was saying. The doctor said he would not recommend the surgery because my dad was too weak, it would be a temporary measure and probably would not help his quality of life. We were all shocked! While staring directly at me, the doctor loudly exclaimed, "If it were my dad, I would take him off the antibiotics and bring him home right now".

We told the doctor that my sister was flying in the following night (Friday evening) and that we wanted to meet together as a family on Saturday at noon to decide. The doctor said that was fine. Just that morning, I was thinking that dad had 306 months of life left and that his acute pancreatitis attack was just a setback that we had to get through until he was stronger - but I was wrong.

How Much Time

I had to find out from the doctor how long my father had to live. I followed the doctor out of the room.

I learned that doctors do not like answering the question: How long does he have to live? I understand that when some people ask this question that they expect an exact answer and get upset if the doctor is wrong. Doctors do not want to be blamed for being wrong and they do not have the ability to predict with certainty when someone will die.

The right way to ask the question is: **Based on your experience, and I won't hold you to it, how long would you expect someone in his condition to live?** I followed the doctor outside my dad's room and asked that very question. The doctor told me 1-2 weeks once his antibiotics were stopped and 2-4 weeks if he was kept on antibiotics. Tears were streaming down my face. I thanked him and took a moment to compose myself before I went back into the room. One week...

When I went back into my dad's room, I asked him if he wanted to have surgery or go home on hospice. At this point in time, he was so weak and could only speak with pauses between words. He fervently told me, "I want to stay here (pause) if I go home (pause) I will be in pain and miserable". I reassured him that he would not be in any pain. Once on hospice, he would be provided with all of the pain medication he needed (that's how it had been explained to me).

We told him that we would take care of him while he was home on hospice and he looked at me and struggled to ask, "Your marriage?" I knew he was implying that taking care of him would somehow interfere with my upcoming marriage and I insisted that taking care of him would in no way affect my marriage. He also was worried about my brother taking time off from his family and my brother told him not to worry. Of course, none of us knew exactly how much time he had left. Even at that moment, dad believed that he had enough life left that caring for him would interfere with our personal lives.

The morphine started to take effect and dad went to sleep. Next to my father's bed, a hospice nurse had left her business card along with a pamphlet. After we left the room, I called her. I told her about our plan to decide on hospice by Saturday afternoon. I told her that dad was frightened about going home and being in pain - I asked that she meet with him to alleviate his fears. At this point, it seemed pretty certain that dad would be on hospice by Saturday. This meant we had to move furniture around to accommodate his hospital bed.

My brother and I left to eat lunch. When we returned to the hospital, dad had a roommate - another cancer patient who was receiving chemotherapy treatments. Dad was visiting with a couple of his friends. He was an outgoing extrovert, so having visitors (even in his weakened state) really cheered him up. When we entered the room, it was apparent that dad was "out of it" mentally. He was so happy and excited. He was no longer speaking with pauses in between his words. He was laughing and kept telling me how amazing it was that I arranged a party for the American Legion at the hospital so that his buddies could come up and visit him. He kept repeating himself.

My brother and I went along with his delusion because he was extremely happy and joyful. Apparently, we did the right thing - if someone is experiencing end of life delirium, it is better to "go along" with the happy delusions instead of contradicting them. The idea is to allow the person to embrace happiness for every moment they have left. My father had been a smart, strong and independent man full of dignity. I felt so helpless watching him become so fragile at the end of his life.

My father's friends left and it was just my dad, my brother and me. From his bed, my dad was intently looking out the window. I asked him if he saw anything. He said he saw flying turkeys. I told him, "yes there are flying turkeys out there" and he laughed. He asked me, "didn't we have a serious conversation earlier with the doctor?" I told him, "Yes, but we didn't have to worry about that right now". We had a pleasant visit with him until he drifted off to sleep again. We left for the night and on our way out I asked the nurse why he had hallucinated. The nurse said that it was probably from either the morphine or his illness.

FRIDAY

Friday morning we woke up and went straight to the hospital. Dad was a bit confused, but no longer hallucinating. He remembered what the doctor had told him about hospice and he began to cry. It was like the reality of everything hit him. He was realizing that he couldn't go hang out with his buddies again - the thing he loved the most. He kept repeating, "I didn't know it (the cancer) was going to get me so soon." I told him I loved him and reassured him that we would keep him pain free. We tried to calm him and told him we were going to bring him home Saturday so he could watch his Yankees games. I never wanted to break down in front of my dad so that he would not spend an ounce of time worrying about me. This was all about him.

Dad then asked me, "How much time do I have?" That shocked me! The doctor gave me an estimate, but I felt it wouldn't be necessary for my dad to know that information. It would only bring him more grief. I told dad that I didn't know, and that he could ask the doctor if he wanted to. Eventually he fell asleep and we went to eat lunch.

At lunch, we talked about dad and hospice. With hospice, they have nurses available at any time for pain medication, but they didn't provide someone in the home 24/7 – one of us would need to stay with dad or we would need to hire a live in. The big question in our minds was what happens after someone dies? We had no idea. Were we supposed to call 911, a non-emergency number or someone else?

After lunch, my brother and I went to meet with a funeral director at the local funeral home. I didn't want to wait until the last minute to do this and had no idea how the funeral process worked. Since dad was divorced, it was up to me to see to it that all of his arrangements were made. We met with the funeral director for an hour and got the process started. It was sad, disheartening and awkward - but it was also a bit of a relief being prepared for when the time came. We learned that once dad had passed away, that all we had to do was call the funeral home and they would retrieve his body.

Friday afternoon, my brother went to pick my sister up at the airport. I went back to the hospital and dad was sleeping. I was looking forward to spending a bit of time alone with him while my brother was out getting my sister. Unfortunately, dad slept the entire time. Right before I was going to leave, his face cringed a bit and he started to shiver. I called for the nurse to put blankets on him. Once he had a bunch of blankets piled onto him, he stopped shivering and was not cringing in pain anymore. I called the hospital late that night and the nurse said dad was comfortable, but that a little earlier he had gotten hot and threw all of his blankets and most of his hospital gown off. That made me chuckle, but I was glad that they were keeping an eye on him.

SATURDAY
Saturday morning - the big day. Our sister had arrived Friday night and we were all staying at dad's house. We rearranged the furniture to make room for the hospital bed near the window so that dad could watch television or watch the deer outside. We surrounded the area with family pictures and set up his favorite reading chair and lamp.

We headed for the hospital and were somewhat joyful that we would be able to bring dad home. When we arrived, my dad instantly recognized my sister and a huge smile appeared on his face. In his weakened state, he kept softly repeating her name. He was so happy to see her, but it was obvious that he was having even more difficult speaking today than the day before.

After his reunion with my sister, he grabbed my hand, looked at me and asked me, "Am I dying?" That broke my heart. I knew he asked me this because he trusted my response. I was straightforward with him and told him, "Yes daddy, you are dying." He nodded his head in the affirmative, squeezed my hand and firmly declared to me that he was "ready to go to my God". He was at peace with dying. He did not get upset because he was ready.

I asked him one final time, did he want to have the surgery or go on hospice. He said he didn't want to have the surgery. I reassured him that he would be comfortable on hospice. I also told him that he didn't have to worry about any of us, and that we would all take care of each other and be fine. He was happy to hear that. He said to us, "All (pause) I want (pause) is your love". We all melted inside, but did our best not to shed any tears. We all held his hand and told him how much we loved him.

We had a pleasant visit with him. He asked for his best friend, and I called his friend to come right away. His friend came to the hospital and they shared their last words with each other. After his friend left, my dad was becoming very sleepy again. I again had told my dad that I loved him. His grip on my hand was so strong. He couldn't respond, but he was able to let out a little smile and winked at me. He closed his eyes to rest.

At about noon, a chaplain came in and gave him the Anointing of the Sick. We were able to wake dad up, but he couldn't speak. He understood that he was receiving the last of the Catholic sacraments and had a huge smile on his face. After the priest left, my brother showed dad that the Yankees had won their game the night before. Dad strained to smile, but was too weak to talk. Afterwards, he drifted off to sleep

Hospice

At about 2 pm, the hospice nurse came to get me because I had Health Care Power of Attorney for my dad. The Healthcare Power of Attorney gave me the authority to sign my dad into hospice.

The hospice nurse informed me that dad's pain was not under control and that he needed to stay in the hospital. I was a bit surprised, but also relieved because dad had been struggling with pain. Every time he was moved by a nurse, he cringed in pain. I didn't want him to suffer at all. When someone is unconscious or in a coma-like state and has pain, they will "communicate" that pain by exhibiting certain body gestures such as cringing. I wasn't familiar with all of those gestures. I was worried that if we brought him home he might give pain signals that we would not recognize as pain.

It was time to officially sign dad into hospice and dad was in a coma-like sleep. Once on hospice, the nurses would remove the IV fluids and antibiotics. He would remain on a morphine drip. I felt like I had to sign the paperwork because it was the most merciful thing I could do for him, yet I felt horrified for "pulling the plug" on someone that I loved. I was crying profusely as I signed the documents, knowing that this was it and it was final. Dad wasn't going to get better and he was dying.

After signing, we went back into dad's room. We watched over him. He did not wake up again and slept all afternoon like he had the prior day. He would cringe in pain when his bed was moved or if his body was moved. Every time he cringed we called the nurse to give him more morphine. Throughout this entire ordeal, I couldn't sleep very much at all. I tried and was only able to sleep about 3 hours each night. I was full of worry, dread and feeling horrible for my dad and his circumstance. The 3 of us stayed overnight with him, but nobody was able to sleep on those uncomfortable hospital chairs.

SUNDAY

Sunday morning, all hope of having him come back with us (consciously) had faded. He didn't wake up at all even after we tried to wake him. He was now in a comatose state. He cringed once in a while in pain and we would immediately get the nurse so he could have extra shots of morphine.

I made phone calls to family members and his friends. People stopped by and spent time with him, which allowed us a little break to go downstairs and eat. The hospice nurses insisted that dad could still hear us even though he could not "wake up". We read to him, played music for him and put on his favorite news channel. We spoke to him as though he was awake. We reminisced about our childhood with him. We told him it was okay for him to go if he wanted to.

Sunday night, the doctors decided to up his morphine dose to 2 mg/hr. At this point, I knew my dad was near death, and it didn't seem productive to move him home on Monday for just a day or two. He couldn't enjoy his home and I was worried about any pain he would experience during the transfer. By Sunday night, he was breathing with his mouth open and his jaw was slacked to the side a bit. I think when he started breathing with his mouth open (instead of shut), he was completely unconscious - but the hospice nurses insisted that we assume he could hear us.

Sunday night, I was able to get a convertible chair/bed from the hospital and I slept overnight in my dad's room. My brother and sister slept at his house due to their bad backs. Finally, after almost a week, I was able to get a good night's sleep because dad's pain appeared to be under control with the increased dosage of morphine. I also felt that mentally, dad was no longer "with us", so I did not have to worry about whether he was panicking inside of his head but unable to wake up to express his fears. It was just a waiting game until his body gave out.

MONDAY

I stayed by dad's side all day on Monday. I read to him and continued to play music and the television news for him. Monday morning my brother took my sister to the airport as she had to get back to her young children.

TUESDAY

When I woke up in dad's room on Tuesday morning, his breathing pattern had changed again. He started to breath, pause, breath, pause... He had a small fever, so they took his vital signs to treat the fever if it got any higher - they wanted him to be comfortable. I told dad I had to leave to go home and take a shower, but that I would be back. For the first time I felt okay leaving him. I hadn't taken a shower since the prior Tuesday. I felt a shower would be good for me and I was now comfortable doing something good for myself. The hospice nurses told us that sometimes people seem to wait until everyone is gone to decide to die. I was giving dad an opportunity if he wanted to take it.

Later that morning, I went to the hospital and dad was still the same. The nurse had noted that dad had mottling at the bottom of his heels. My brother and I played some soft music for him on the hospital television. Later that afternoon, my brother and I both had small headaches and rested in our chairs.

A knock on the door woke me up from my 10 minute cat nap. A chaplain had walked in and asked how we were doing. We said we were fine. I looked at dad and his breathing had changed dramatically in just 10 minutes. The pauses between his breaths were now 30 seconds long. I mentioned that to the chaplain and the chaplain said that dying people had breathing rates that could increase, then slowdown, then increase again. Not one minute later, and dad's breaths became just tiny puffs of air about a minute apart. The chaplain saw this and said he would get the nurses. After about 5 of these tiny puffs, dad took his last tiny puff of air and stopped breathing. It was over. He was gone. I gave him a kiss and said I was proud of him.

What Caused My Father's Death

Pancreatic cancer was the cause of my father's death, but we will never know exactly how it caused his death. It could have been that the acute pancreatitis caused septic shock and shut his organs down. It could have been that the cancer itself weakened his body so much that his entire body decided to shut down. It could have been an uncontrolled infection in the bile duct (cholangitis) that carried elsewhere in his body that caused his body to shut down. I later found out that he also had a very infected gallbladder that had air inside of it (the air was the byproduct of bacteria taking it over) and this could have caused sepsis. Regardless of the exact cause, it was ultimately pancreatic cancer that took his life.

The following information consists of my research on pancreatic cancer. When someone is diagnosed with cancer, the doctors don't have time to go over all of the information in this book. They use their knowledge of the disease to provide the most immediate diagnostic treatment options so that the patient can decide what to do next. It seems as though pamphlets, brochures and websites only give partial information - sometimes very general information.

When faced with cancer, many don't have any idea what is going to happen and how to approach cancer diagnostics and treatment. Arming yourself with knowledge can help you know what to expect, what your options are, how to speak more intelligently with your doctors, how to advocate for yourself or loved ones and how to know if you are receiving substandard care. This information can help you make the best choices according to the situation.

As a family member, it was frustrating not having a single "go to" resource to acquire the information I needed to feel informed and confident that my father was receiving the proper treatment. This cancer hit so quickly that I didn't have the time to research and process all of the information that I needed to be prepared. Hopefully, this book will provide others more confidence when faced with pancreatic cancer.

Of course, none of this is intended as medical advice and should not be relied upon as such. Also, by the time you read this book, some of this information may be out of date, so it is encouraged that you talk to your doctors and do your own research as well.

CHAPTER TWO

WHAT IS PANCREATIC CANCER

The Pancreas

The pancreas is about 6 inches long, functions as a glandular organ, looks like a small banana and is located behind the stomach. It produces digestive enzymes that are emptied out into the small intestines to aid in digestion. The pancreas also produces insulin. Because of its location behind the stomach, it is very difficult to see pancreatic tumors in a regular CT scan. With suspected cases of pancreatic cancer, it is highly recommended that a **3 phase helical pancreatic protocol CT scan with contrast** be performed.

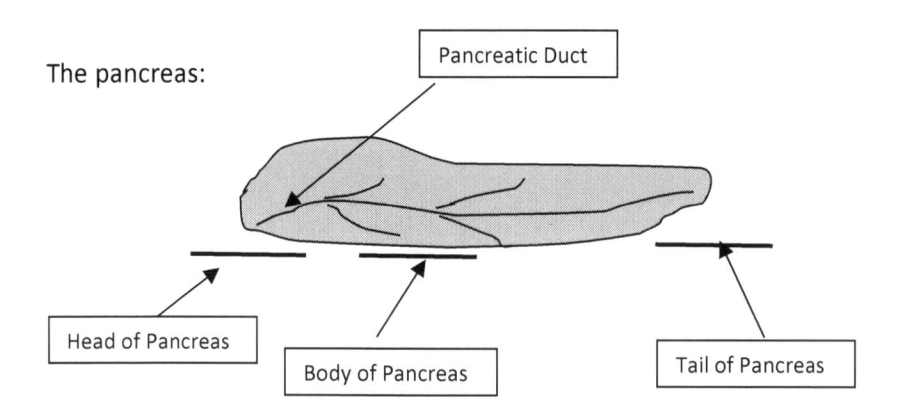

The pancreas:

- Pancreatic Duct
- Head of Pancreas
- Body of Pancreas
- Tail of Pancreas

The Pancreas makes digestive enzymes which flow down the pancreatic duct, into the common bile duct and then finally into the small intestines where it aids in food digestion.

The gastrointestinal area looks like this:

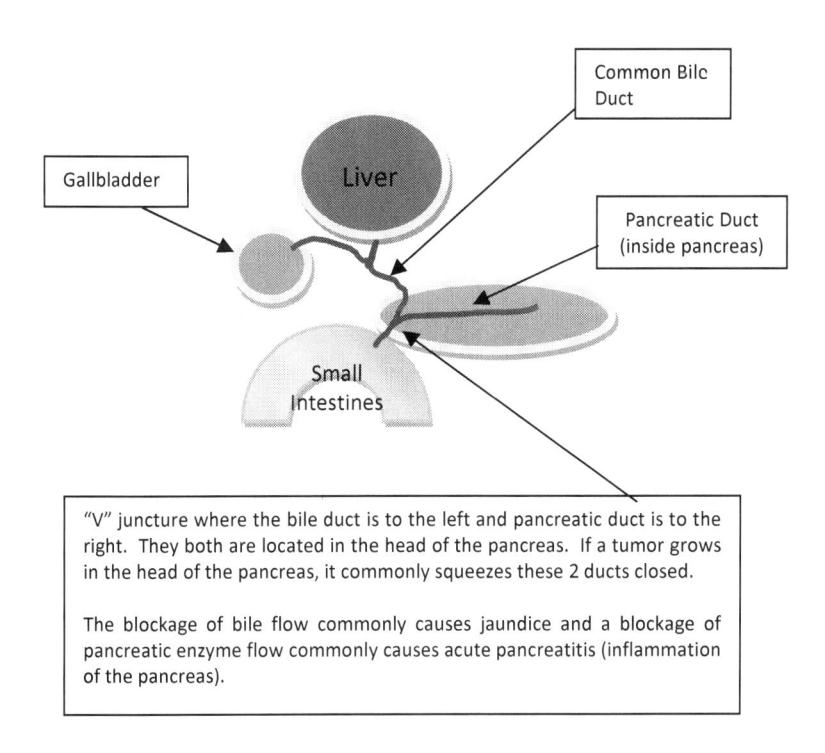

[Diagram showing Gallbladder, Liver, Common Bile Duct, Pancreatic Duct (inside pancreas), and Small Intestines]

"V" juncture where the bile duct is to the left and pancreatic duct is to the right. They both are located in the head of the pancreas. If a tumor grows in the head of the pancreas, it commonly squeezes these 2 ducts closed.

The blockage of bile flow commonly causes jaundice and a blockage of pancreatic enzyme flow commonly causes acute pancreatitis (inflammation of the pancreas).

The liver manufactures bile and sends it over to the gallbladder. Bile aids in digesting fats. When we eat, the gallbladder pumps bile through the common bile duct into the small intestines to aid in digestion.

The pancreas manufactures special enzymes which aid in digestion. As you can see in the diagram, the common bile duct passes through the head of the pancreas. At the "V" juncture within the pancreas, the pancreatic duct sends its digestive enzymes into the bile duct and mixes with the bile. This mixture of bile and pancreatic enzymes is dumped into the small intestines and helps the body to digest the food we eat. If a tumor forms in the head of the pancreas, then that tumor can easily press on and narrow (stricture) both the pancreatic duct and bile duct (aka the "Double Duct Sign").

Pancreatic Cancer

There are different types of pancreatic cancer, but most people (85-90%) diagnosed with pancreatic cancer get **Pancreatic Adenocarcinoma** - a cancerous tumor that grows in the head of the pancreas.

Our bodies are made up of many cells. Cells usually die off and new cells replace the ones that die. A cancer is a cell that divides and replicates itself, but never dies off. Eventually, the growing clump of cancer cells form a tumor. The tumor grows and interferes with the function of organs. Pancreatic cancer tumors can grow large enough to block the bile duct, pancreatic duct and the small intestines.

Humans can live without their pancreas as pancreatic digestive enzymes can be replaced in pill form. Usually, by the time pancreatic cancer is discovered, the cancerous tumor cells have metastasized (moved) to other locations in the body and tumors have started to grow in other organs (like the liver).

Typically, those with pancreatic cancer end up dying of liver failure as metastasized tumors cause the liver to fail. Unfortunately, humans cannot live without a functioning liver. The liver performs too many important intricate functions which we cannot replicate with medical devices or medicine.

In my dad's case, the tumor pressed down on his pancreatic duct and common bile duct (aka Double Duct Sign). Due to the narrowing of these ducts, a gallstone got stuck in the stricture of the common bile duct and blocked the bile from entering the intestines. Also, my dad's pancreatic duct narrowed and his pancreatic enzymes could not properly drain into the common bile duct. As a result, my dad suffered from jaundice and had attacks of acute pancreatitis. He did not have treatment options. His original bile duct stent failed, he had a severely infected gallbladder, he probably had an infected bile duct (cholangitis) and he had severe pancreatitis. If he had attempted to have a bile duct bypass operation where a bag would be put on the exterior of his body to drain the bile, then he probably would have passed away on the operating table.

CHAPTER THREE

SYMPTOMS OF PANCREATIC CANCER

Pancreatic cancer is one of the deadliest cancers because:

1. The cancer often doesn't cause symptoms until it has progressed to a point where the cancer has metastasized or it has wrapped itself around vital vessels which make removing it impossible.

2. The earliest symptoms are so non-descript, that they can be easily mistaken for more common and less serious ailments. By the time the symptoms are connected to pancreatic cancer - the cancer has already spread.

3. It is more difficult for medical testing to visualize the pancreas because it is hidden behind the stomach - so tumors don't always show up on regular CT scans or other tests. Pancreatic cancers are normally not palpable (able to be felt by pressing the hand down onto the skin).

Tumors are classified as either noncancerous (benign) or cancerous (malignant). The common way to confirm a diagnosis of cancer is to stick a needle directly into the tumor and test the cells for malignancy. Most doctors do NOT want to do a needle biopsy for suspected pancreatic cancer because a needle biopsy can cause cancer cells to break off of the tumor and metastasize elsewhere in the body. As a result, many pancreatic cancer patients never receive a confirmed "positive" biopsy of their pancreatic cancer. Usually blood tests with liver panel screening, CA19-9 blood marker screening, visualizing the tumor on scans and tracking the growth rate of the tumor along with presenting symptoms are enough to diagnose pancreatic cancer.

In the case of my father, he first presented with painless jaundice and no itchiness. They thought his bile duct was blocked by a simple gallstone. It is not unusual for a small gallstone to pass down the bile duct and out of the digestive system without causing pain, but when a **sizeable** *gallstone does get stuck in the bile duct, it usually causes* **pain** *as it scrapes the sides of the bile duct on its way down the duct. It appears that my father had a small gallstone that was making its way painlessly down the bile duct when it got stuck due to the narrowing of the bile duct and that is why he did not feel any pain.*

When the surgeon went inside my father's bile duct with a scope, he saw that my father had the "double duct sign" which was a narrowing of both the bile duct and pancreatic duct. The "Double Duct Sign" is a pretty good indication that pancreatic cancer is present. The doctor ordered 2 regular CT scans for my father – and the doctor was never able to visualize the tumor. I would not be surprised if the specialist who originally removed the gallstone and placed the stent in the bile duct was able to see a tiny tumor when my father had the ERCP performed – but I never was able to get a copy of those medical records. My father died so quickly that he never had a special pancreatic protocol CT scan which probably would have enabled doctors to identify and stage the tumor.

Symptoms of Pancreatic Cancer

Any of these symptoms may occur together, in combination or alone. Symptoms may come and go as well. The most common symptoms are back pain along with weight loss and/or jaundice.

Pain
- In abdomen and/or back

Fatigue
- Tired and/or weakness
- Getting up Later and/or Sleeping More Often

Jaundice (Especially Painless Jaundice)
- Dark Urine
- Yellow skin or eyes
- Clay colored stools
- Itchy skin

Fluid in Abdomen (Ascites)
- Feeling of Fullness
- Feeling of Fluid Swishing Around in Abdomen
- Unusually Distended Abdomen (Belly Sticks Out)

Swelling
- Painful swelling of arm or leg (due to blood clot)

Gastrointestinal Complaints
- Bloating - Sense of Fullness in Stomach
- Burning in stomach
- Nausea
- Loss of Appetite
- Vomiting
- Chills
- Fever
- Unexplained Weight Loss
- Floating Stools with Bad Odor or Unusual Color

Enlarged Lymph Nodes

Development of Type 2 Diabetes
(Generally occurs with rarer forms of pancreatic cancer occurring in tail of pancreas where insulin is produced)

Elevated Liver Enzymes with Routine Blood Tests

Possible Mass Felt in Abdomen

CHAPTER FOUR

TESTING FOR PANCREATIC CANCER

There are no screening tests for the early detection of pancreatic cancer. For example, a mammography is a screening test designed to provide early detection of breast cancer. Stool tests are designed to provide early detection for colon cancer. There have been some companies who are working on a urine or blood test to screen for early stage pancreatic cancer, but none have finished trials and been approved by the FDA. It is hoped that within 10 years there will be a screening test available for the early detection of pancreatic cancer.

When Pancreatic Cancer is Suspected Due to Presenting Symptoms and Bloodwork, the Following Tests Are Used:

Ultrasound
Ultrasound technology uses harmless waves that bounce off of organs and form a picture. Ultrasound can be used to locate some pancreatic cancers.

3 Phase Helical Pancreatic Protocol CT Scan With Contrast
A CT scan uses X-Rays to form a picture. It is vital that if pancreatic cancer is suspected, that the patient be given a 3 Phase Helical Pancreatic Protocol CT Scan as soon as possible for staging (which can determine the best treatment protocol). A regular CT scan is not good enough at detecting many pancreatic cancers. The 3 Phase CT is different from a regular CT: Contrast (a type of radiation) is used and the pictures taken (3mm slices) are thinner than a regular CT scan pictures (5mm-6mm slices). As the contrast travels through your body it

"highlights" certain body structures first - then, as it makes its way through organs it starts to highlight other body structures. So, depending on what type of contrast used and the exact time that certain pictures are taken – doctors can get a pretty good look at the pancreas and its surrounding structures.

MRI
An MRI uses magnetic waves to form a picture and can locate some pancreatic cancers. It cannot be used on some patients (my dad could not have an MRI due to his pacemaker).

PET Scan
PET Scans use a contrast that is absorbed by cancerous tumors. PET scans are good for detecting the spread of cancer.

Biopsy
A tumor (overgrowth of cells) can be malignant or benign. With a benign tumor, the tumor cells are not programmed to grow uncontrollably and usually the tumor will not interfere with the function of an organ. With a malignant tumor, the tumor cells are programmed to continuously multiply and will keep spreading until they interfere with the function of an organ unless they are removed or killed. A biopsy, or taking a sample of the actual tumor, is the only way to diagnose with certainty that a specific tumor is malignant or benign. Recovering cancerous cells from body fluids and/or metastasized tumors that are easier to reach can also aid in diagnosis.

Doctors usually do not biopsy pancreatic tumors because they are very difficult to reach. Additionally, pancreatic cancer is much more prone to metastasis than other types of cancerous tumors. If you break a piece of bread in half, you will inevitably cause crumbs to fall to the counter. Similarly, if a sharp instrument is used to pierce and remove a piece of pancreatic cancer tumor, then microscopic pancreatic cancer cells will also fall off into the body which can cause the cancer to spread (metastasis).

For those with pancreatic cancer a brush biopsy is commonly performed in the bile duct during an ERCP for pancreatic cancer and/or during stent placement after the bile duct has become blocked. A surgeon uses a tiny brush to brush cells off of the inner bile duct wall where a stricture is occurring. These cells are then tested for malignancy. In addition, during this procedure, a surgeon may also collect pancreatic juices from the pancreatic duct and examine the juice for the presence of microscopic pancreatic cancer cells.

My dad had an ERCP, where a tube was pushed down his throat, into the stomach, into the small intestines and up the common bile duct. While in the bile duct, the doctors were able to place a stent to open his bile duct back up (relieving the jaundice) and to also take a brush biopsy of the inside of the bile duct for cancer cells. With a brush biopsy, they take a brush and gently brush the site being tested and then send the cells that are collected to a lab to find out if the cells are cancerous or not. My father did not have cancerous cells in his bile duct - he had what are called "atypical cells". This indicated that the pancreatic cancer tumor had not invaded the bile duct; instead, the tumor was only putting pressure on the bile duct to make it squeeze shut.

*** NOTE: A negative brush biopsy of the inner common bile duct does not mean that someone does not have pancreatic cancer - it only means that no cancerous cells were found in the bile duct itself.

Something that frustrated me was that my dad's primary care physician told me and my dad that the bile duct biopsy was positive for pancreatic cancer. My dad's surgeon told me that the brush biopsy was negative for pancreatic cancer cells, but it was positive for "atypical cells" (possibly pre-cancerous). I cannot explain why I received 2 different medical conclusions for the single brush biopsy that my father had. When people do not have a definitive answer as to what is "wrong", it can cause stress. I can only surmise that my father's primary care physician knew my dad had pancreatic cancer and just wanted to confirm the biopsy as being positive so that we would feel less stress and uncertainty over what was happening to my dad.

CHAPTER FIVE

STATISTICS AND STAGING OF PANCREATIC CANCER

WHO GETS PANCREATIC CANCER

About 50,000 people per year in the U.S. are diagnosed with pancreatic cancer with almost a 50/50 split between men and women - with men being diagnosed with it a little more often. When compared to the general population, black males have a bit of a higher chance of getting it and Asian women having a little bit of a lower chance of getting it. There are different types of pancreatic cancer, but most people who get it (95%) are diagnosed with pancreatic Adenocarcinoma - cancer in the head of the Pancreas. The other 5% have pancreatic cancer in the neck, body or tail of the Pancreas. The median age of diagnosis is 71 years old (my dad was 85). If immediate family members are diagnosed with pancreatic cancer, you will be more likely to get it; however, the majority of people diagnosed with pancreatic cancer have no family members who have had it. 50% of people diagnosed with pancreatic cancer are overweight or obese and up to 80% have type 2 diabetes or are insulin resistant.

Age group breakdown

Under 20 Years of Age	0.1%
20-34 Years of Age	0.5%
35-44 Years of Age	2.1%
45-54 Years of Age	9.2%
55-64 Years of Age	21.9%
65-74 Years of Age	26.8%
74-84 Years of Age	26.1%
Over 84 Years of Age	13.5%

Staging of pancreatic Cancer

Stage 0
Tumor confined to top layers of pancreatic duct and has not invaded deeper tissues. It has not spread to other areas.

Stage 1A
Tumor confined to pancreas and is 2 cm across or smaller. It has not spread to other areas.

Stage 1B
Tumor is confined to pancreas and is larger than 2 cm across. It has not spread to other areas.

Stage 2A
Tumor is growing outside of pancreas but not into major blood vessels or nerves. It has not spread to other areas.

Stage 2B
Tumor is either confined or growing outside the pancreas but not into major blood vessels or nerves. It HAS spread to nearby lymph nodes.

Stage 3: Tumor is growing outside pancreas into nearby major blood vessels or nerves. It may or may not have spread to nearby lymph nodes, but it has not spread to distant sites.

Stage 4: The tumor has spread to distant sites.

At the Time of Diagnosis, Approximately:
- 9% have a tumor confined to the pancreas
- 28% have a tumor that has spread to the lymph nodes
- 53% have a Stage 4 tumor that has spread to distant sites
- 10% have an unknown stage

Note: My father's stage was unknown and never will be known. He died so quick he never even had a chance to have it staged. Generally, people who have painless jaundice as the first symptom have a TINY bit of a better chance of long term survival because painless jaundice is usually associated with the pancreatic cancer having been caught at an earlier

stage (thus these patients have a higher chance of qualifying for surgery).

5 Year Survival rate broken down by stage for Adenocarcinoma (Cancer in Head of Pancreas)

Stage 1A	14%
Stage 1B	12%
Stage IIA	7%
Stage IIB	5%
Stage III	3%
Stage IV	1%

General Prognosis: About 20% of people diagnosed with pancreatic cancer survive a year. Most will succumb to the cancer within 3-6 months. From the time he had jaundice, my father passed away within 30 days. From the time of his "official" diagnosis, he passed in 2 weeks and 2 days.

A Cure
The only cure for pancreatic cancer is to surgically remove it. Only about 15%-20% of people diagnosed with pancreatic cancer will qualify for surgery. Of those who qualify for surgery - about 30% will have their surgery aborted once they are on the operating table and opened up because the surgeons will find either that the cancer has metastasized, find evidence of ascites (which generally means death is very near), or find that the tumor has grown too close to major structures (it is unresectable).

Chemotherapy and radiation do not cure pancreatic cancer, but they are usually offered to those diagnosed with pancreatic cancer because they tend to slow the progression of the cancer, add a few more months of life and improve the quality of life left. Even those who have surgery are likely to have a recurrence over a five year period (about 85%). Recurrence happens because very early on in the disease process, pancreatic cancer cells tend to migrate and "hide out" within body. These microscopic cells eventually grow cancerous tumors in other organs (i.e., liver).

Whipple Surgery - Who Qualifies

The primary surgery used for pancreatic cancer removal is called the "Whipple Surgery" which was developed by Dr. Allen Whipple in 1935. Mortality for the surgery is about 4% if the surgery is performed at a cancer center where a high volume of Whipple Surgeries are performed - otherwise, the mortality rate is closer to 16%. Age alone is not a barrier for having the Whipple Surgery. **NOTE: IF YOU QUALIFY FOR THE SURGERY, THEN HAVE THE SURGERY AT A CENTER THAT PERFORMS AT LEAST 20 WHIPPLE OPERATIONS A YEAR (20+ IS CONSIDERED "HIGH VOLUME").**

Pancreatic cancer is generally considered **resectable** if the surgeon believes the entire cancer can be removed. Often, the tumor wraps itself around the superior mesenteric artery and vein (which run through the pancreas) and cannot be removed although the tumor itself is confined to the pancreas (aka Locally Advanced Cancer).

A minority of Stage 3 cancers are considered to be "borderline resectable". If chemo and radiation shrink the tumor to the point that the removal of the tumor no longer compromises the superior mesenteric artery and vein, then surgery will be attempted. For cancer that has spread, surgery might be an option if it is used to relieve symptoms.

Self-Advocacy – 3 Levels of Fight

Once pancreatic cancer is suspected, diagnosed and staged - it is important for each patient to decide for himself if he wants to be passive, moderately aggressive or highly aggressive in fighting the cancer.

Passive: Being passive means either that the patient allows the doctors lead the treatment plan or the patient refuses all treatment except palliative care and/or hospice.

Moderately Aggressive: Being moderately aggressive means that the patient will let the doctors mostly lead, but the patient will do research about their condition and speak up with questions or about the direction the patient wants the treatment to take.

Highly Aggressive: Being highly aggressive means that the patient will fight tooth and nail to qualify for the Whipple surgery, the patient will seek out oncologists who agree with and support very aggressive treatment and the patient will do extensive research to ensure that he has enough information to fight this cancer with everything he has got.

There is no wrong decision, but those with pancreatic cancer should be aware that they have a choice in their treatment - and their decision on how aggressive to be should be made as quickly as possible once pancreatic Cancer is **suspected**. Although family members may want a different level of aggression than the patient - the patient's decision on how aggressive he or she wants to be should be respected by all well-meaning friends, family and treating physicians.

My dad took a laid back approach to his cancer diagnosis. He was completely unaware of most of the information that I have written in this book. He did not realize that this cancer could take him in a matter of a few weeks (I didn't either). His doctors were very lackadaisical in taking their time on returning the biopsy results, telling him he didn't qualify for treatment, not preparing him ahead of time for preventing acute pancreatitis or giving him medications ahead of time for pain, nausea and vomiting. I think my father should have had a palliative care consultation during his first hospitalization when they highly suspected pancreatic cancer - so that he might have been able to prevent the 2 bouts of acute pancreatitis and maybe have lived a little longer with less discomfort.

On his death bed, prior to being at peace with his impending death - he kept saying, "I didn't know this would get me so quick." When he was first told he probably had pancreatic cancer, I didn't push him or reveal to him much of anything about the cancer. It became very obvious very quickly that he couldn't have any treatment for it, so what was the point in forcing information on him and scaring him. If he wanted to know more information about the cancer, he could have asked his doctor, asked me questions or read the book that I had offered.

He was so weak from his hospitalizations and the cancer itself that he needed to use all of his strength to recover from those hospitalizations. He did not have the mental strength to even begin to cope with being diagnosed with pancreatic cancer. As a supportive family member, it was my duty to let him lead his treatment. I would have only caused him a lot of stress if I had forced information on him, forced him to eat, forced him to see an oncologist or forced him to submit to various treatments.

Despite what happened to my father, there are many people diagnosed with pancreatic cancer who are able to prolong their life or have a decent quality of life with various treatments.

CHAPTER SIX

GAME PLAN FOR PANCREATIC CANCER

1. **PRIMARY CARE PHYSICIAN**:
Most people have a health concern, visit their primary care physician for help, and their primary care physician will run tests to try to diagnose the problem. In the case of pancreatic cancer, a primary care physician will suspect pancreatic cancer due to a combination of symptoms and bloodwork results. Primary care physicians do not specialize in treating cancer; therefore, once a physician tells you he suspects pancreatic cancer it is vital that you see a medical oncologist (a doctor who specializes in cancer) as soon as possible to have the cancer diagnosis confirmed, to have the cancer staged and to have the cancer treated.

2. **MEDICAL ONCOLOGIST**:
As soon as a patient with pancreatic cancer is symptomatic, pancreatic cancer is an EXTREMELY QUICK progressing disease. If pancreatic cancer is suspected, get a confirmed diagnosis as soon as possible with the special Pancreatic Protocol CT Scan. Even if you ultimately decide to be Passive in your treatment; timewise, it's REALLY important to be AGGRESSIVE with getting the cancer **diagnosed and staged** in order to maximize treatment options and maximize the timeframe to exercise the treatment options you choose.

As soon as pancreatic cancer is suspected – get a referral to a medical oncologist and visit a medical oncologist right away. Find out the type of pancreatic cancer (most people have cancer in the head of the Pancreas). You may need to "push" the issue and not "settle" for waiting 1-3 weeks until they can "fit you in" for a scan or to see an oncologist.

During my father's episode, I had read that finding an oncologist who specializes in pancreatic cancer was important. There were no specialists in my area and my dad was too weak to travel. I later learned that visiting a regular medical oncologist was more important than seeing a specialist in order to get the cancer diagnosis confirmed and staged as soon as possible. You can always have a regular medical oncologist refer you to a specialist or ask him to consult with a specialist. For example, if it takes 3 weeks to get an appointment with a specialist and only 3 days to get an appointment with a medical oncologist who doesn't specialize in pancreatic cancer – your best bet is to see the medical oncologist who does not specialize in order to get the cancer diagnosed and staged as soon as possible.

To make things go "faster", as soon as you hear from your primary care physician that cancer may be suspected, begin calling various medical oncologist offices in order to get an appoint with a medical oncologist as soon as possible. Find out who has the earliest appointment available and make that appointment. Tell the receptionists at the medical oncologist's offices that you need an appointment as soon as possible because pancreatic cancer is suspected. Once you have the appointment, ask your doctor for a referral to the medical oncologist that you made an appointment with.

In my father's case, he was too weak, frail and in poor health to even consider going to another doctor's appointment. In his circumstance it would have been much better if he had seen a palliative care doctor in the hospital who could have helped him have a much better quality of life during his last month.

3. **TREAT SYMPTOMS**:

   Treat the immediate symptoms as soon as possible (i.e., jaundice, pain, nausea, vomiting). The sooner the symptoms are treated, the better chance the patient has of maintaining physical strength. Patients who are overall healthier are more likely to qualify for future chemo, radiation and surgery. Untreated symptoms take a toll on the body and poor physical health can disqualify patients for cancer treatments. Ask your medical oncologist to set you up with a TEAM of doctors who can help you treat the cancer and the symptoms. This team should include a surgical oncologist to determine if curative surgery is possible or for surgery to treat symptoms as they arise, a palliative care specialist (pain medications) and nutritionist (to keep you in optimal health).

4. **TREATMENT PLAN**:

   Formulate a written treatment plan with your team of doctors taking into consideration how aggressive you wish to be in fighting the cancer. Tell your doctors how passive or aggressive you want to be with your treatment. As a reminder, if survival is your goal and you want aggressive treatment, you may need to "shop" around until you find a doctor who will support your goals. Some surgical oncologists are more aggressive than others and will agree to do the Whipple Surgery when most other surgical oncologists refuse to do so. If your pancreatic cancer is "borderline resectable" – you may need to fight to have the Whipple Surgery performed.

5. **<u>PREVENTATIVE CARE</u>:**

    Have your team of doctors also provide you with a supply of medications you will need ahead of time. Many times this care is done by a Palliative Care Doctor. He can provide:
    - Pain medications
    - Break-Through Pain Medications (an additional pain medication prescribed in case the pain becomes so bad that the regularly prescribed pain medication does not work). If you find yourself taking the break-through pain medication more frequently over time, then ask your doctor for a stronger dose or a different type of regular pain medication.
    - Anti-nausea Medications
    - Anti-vomiting Medications

    Remember, untreated pain is unnecessary. No one needs to live with pain. Pancreatic cancer patients do not need to worry about addiction to pain medications. Untreated pain causes the stress hormones to rise within the patient's body – elevated stress hormones can harm the cancer patient in numerous ways.

    We are all used to getting sick with something, and then seeing a doctor for relief. With pancreatic cancer, the approach is MUCH different. With pancreatic cancer, most people will eventually have pain and vomiting. With chemotherapy, most people will have reactions to it. Instead of waiting until symptoms like pain and vomiting occur and THEN visiting a doctor; a palliative care physician will prescribe medications ahead of time so that people with pancreatic cancer can address those symptoms at home without having to go see a doctor each time a symptom occurs.

In my dad's case, if he had visited with a palliative care doctor, he could have had medication at home for the nausea, vomiting and pain when he was struck with acute pancreatitis. He might not have had to spend an entire night vomiting if he had known that a larger meal could cause acute pancreatitis. If we had the information that a palliative care physician could have provided us with, we might have been able to prevent the acute pancreatitis.

6. **NUTRITIONIST**:

Meet with a nutritionist who specializes in cancer nutrition. Those with cancer usually need to increase their calorie intake; however, those with a narrowed pancreatic duct may need to eat in very special ways to prevent acute pancreatitis. Some cancer patients may need assistance in putting on weight to help them qualify for treatments.

My dad was not told that due to his narrowed pancreatic duct, he should have been eating many tiny meals so as not to cause his pancreatic juices to back up in his pancreas and cause acute pancreatitis. He spent 2 hospitalizations in severe pain with nausea and vomiting due to acute pancreatitis. Acute pancreatitis can cause death in 25% of patients who have it.

7. **PSYCHOLOGIST**:

Being diagnosed with cancer can be scary and traumatic. It is recommended to have at least one meeting with a psychologist who specializes in working with cancer patients to help deal with the diagnosis, worries, depression and other issues that may come up. Having a healthy mindset can help make treatments more effective.

8. **<u>FAMILY GAME PLAN</u>**:

Cancer patients need the support of friends and family. My dad was too weak to cook, clean and do laundry. I took care of him after each hospitalization. I had planned to be his primary caretaker once he was home on hospice - with visiting nurses and home health aides coming part time to assist. My dad didn't have an opportunity to make many decisions in his treatment because he was too weak, too sick and spent most of his last month in a hospital. Fortunately, most people diagnosed with pancreatic Cancer have a bit more time than we did to prepare and make decisions.

Some questions to ask at a family meeting:
1. Can someone live with the patient while they receive treatment?
2. Who can bring the patient to and from various medical appointments?
3. Does the patient need financial assistance to live or take care of medical costs (copays, food, etc...)?
4. Can someone live with the patient if they go into hospice at home?
5. Can people take turns living with and/or caring for the patient?
6. Can a schedule be made to ensure someone is always there with the patient?
7. Will home health aides need to be hired?
8. Does the patient have long term healthcare insurance to help pay for a live-in?
9. Does the patient qualify for any programs to help?
10. Are there free services available for transportation to appointments?
11. How can social services help?
12. How will respite (breaks) be arranged for family members or friends who are living with the patient?

Family Interaction with the Patient

It's vital for the patient with cancer to be the one to LEAD his family and friends in this process. It does NOT help a cancer patient to have his family trying to force information about the cancer onto him, to force him into treatment, or to force food down his throat by using guilt, anger or any other type of manipulation. Cancer patients always need to be in complete control of their own illness and treatment and it is important that family members acknowledge and recognize that.

CANCER PATIENT'S RIGHTS:

Every cancer patient has rights that must be respected by doctors, family members and friends:

1. It is a cancer patient's RIGHT whether or not they WANT to know their prognosis. Family members and friends should NEVER tell a cancer patient what their prognosis is. ONLY a medical doctor who is familiar with the patient's specific medical history and diagnosis can communicate that to a patient. Most doctors will respect the cancer patient's rights and ASK if the cancer patient wants to know their prognosis before sharing that information with a cancer patient.

2. It is a cancer patient's RIGHT to have full access to all of their medical records and information so that they can make the most informed decision on their treatment. Typically, during a doctor visit, the doctor will give a very brief synopsis on what is occurring and then give the patient treatment options. The treating doctor does not normally provide copies of medical records to the patient and go over what the medical records mean. It is a patient's right to be able to see his medical records and have questions about his medical records and condition answered in full so that he can make an informed decision. This may mean that the patient and/or family members that the patient relies upon may need to pressure the doctor for access to the medical records.

3. It is a cancer patient's RIGHT to share what information they WANT to share with friends and family about their illness. Some cancer patient's want only

a couple of family members to know about their illness and do not want everyone else to know about it. If a cancer patient shares with you that they have cancer, it is a violation of that person's rights if you tell others about the diagnosis without the cancer patient's permission to do so. It is a violation of that person's rights to post announcements on Facebook or the internet about their diagnosis without permission. It is a violation of that person's rights to start a fundraiser without their permission. It is a violation of that person's rights to share the information with church members, employers, family, friends or neighbors. Generally speaking, cancer patients usually want to be the ones to tell people about their condition and they do not want other people doing this for them.

4. It is a cancer patient's RIGHT not to have family members and friends constantly asking personal questions. Well-meaning family members and friends should NEVER ask the cancer patient "What did the doctor say?" or "what were your test results?" or "Are you going to have chemotherapy?" or "Have you experienced pain or vomiting?" Instead, the cancer patient should be allowed to share what they feel comfortable about sharing.

5. It is a cancer patient's RIGHT to choose their treatment without being confronted by others. If a cancer patient chooses NOT to have surgery or chemotherapy, then well-meaning family members and friends need to 100% support that decision instead of arguing with the patient or pleading with the patient to take treatment.

6. It is a cancer patient's RIGHT to eat or not to eat. It can be alarming for friends and family watch a cancer patient "waste away"; however, it is extremely harmful to try to force a cancer patient to eat. Again, friends and family are not doctors and if they are worried they can offer to bring the patient to a nutritionist if the patient chooses to see one – other than that, friends and family should not make any comments about a cancer patient's weight, what a cancer patient eats or how much a cancer patient eats. The gastrointestinal system is one of the first systems to shut down when a person is getting closer to death. In response to this preparation for death, the appetite of a cancer patient will decrease over time. It is extremely harmful to try to force a cancer patient to eat when this process is occurring. This is why only a doctor and/or nutritionist who specializes in treating cancer patients should give advice to the cancer patient on weight, food and food intake.

7. It is a cancer patient's RIGHT to be free from having to hear comments about their appearance. Family members and friends should NEVER make comments to a cancer patient about their appearance – whether it be about their hair, weight, skin tone, skin appearance or overall appearance. It is silly to tell a cancer patient that they look "great" and it is insulting to tell a cancer patient that they look "awful". Cancer patients already know how they look and it is important for family members and friends to refrain from making any comments about their appearance.

8. It is a cancer patient's RIGHT to be free from drama. Every friend and family member should do their best NOT to involve the cancer patient in anything negative. Negative news or negative drama that affects the cancer patient

can cause distress. Elevated stress hormones can physically HARM a cancer patient. If "Uncle Roger" cheated on "Aunt Linda", the cancer patient doesn't need to know about it. If "Cousin Jonny" got hit by a car, the cancer patient doesn't need to know about it. If "Todd" and "Linda" are getting a divorce, the cancer patient doesn't need to know about it. Some family members and friends find it a hobby to torment others. If a family member has historically given the cancer patient a hard time, then communication with that family member should be discontinued for as long as the cancer patient has cancer.

9. It is a cancer patient's RIGHT to control his or her own visitation schedule. Some cancer patients do not want ANYONE to visit. Some cancer patients want as many people to visit them as possible. Some cancer patients only want certain people to visit at certain times of the day or on certain days of the week. A cancer patient who was outgoing and loved people prior to diagnosis may become more reclusive.

It's also important to recognize that cancer is a whole body illness. A person who was formerly at the center stage when it came to family drama and gossip may not have the emotional or physical ability to handle the drama like she did before the diagnosis. A person who loved being around the 10 grandkids before the diagnosis may no longer be able to physically or emotionally handle having the 10 grandkids around her now. It is a cancer patient's RIGHT to control who visits them and when.

Well-meaning friends and family members should never "drop by" unless invited. Those who are invited should never bring others with them without those specific people being invited as well. For example, if "Suzie" was invited, then she should not bring her 3 kids along with her unless they were specifically invited as well. Small children can cause stress to cancer patients.

Some patients will have chemotherapy or radiation scheduled on certain days of the week and do not want visitors on those days. Some patients want specific people to come over after chemo/radiation treatment so that they can get assistance with the vomiting and nausea. It is always up to the cancer patient to choose who visits and when.

It's important for family members and loved ones to recognize that they may be taking their anger and/or fears out on their sick relative and that they may need therapeutic support themselves. If friends or family members find themselves trying to control the actions of the cancer patient (i.e., forcing them to eat or violating any of the rights of the cancer patient as listed above), then that person should no longer be allowed to interact with the cancer patient until they get therapeutic services that help them learn how to handle a friend or family member who has cancer.

When my dad was diagnosed, I asked him if he wanted to see an oncologist. He said he was too weak at that time. I didn't badger him into seeing one (although I really wanted him to see one right away). Prior to his doctor appointment for the biopsy results, I purchased a book on pancreatic cancer. I nonchalantly told my dad that I had the book and if he wanted to read to be more informed about pancreatic cancer before his doctor appointment to just ask me for it. He never asked for it and I never brought it up again.

When it came to food and drink, I let my dad lead me on what he wanted to eat and drink. I never told him what he should or shouldn't be eating.

Although I researched pancreatic Cancer on the internet and knew he probably had a short time span left (3-6 months is typical), I didn't tell my dad what I had read. I was not his doctor and did not know what his specific medical prognosis was. I'm glad that I respected my father's rights as a cancer patient because all that the information would have done would be to have frightened him. As family members and friends, it's our duty to be supportive of what the patient WANTS and NEEDS and DESIRES - not to try to tell the patient what to do. From personal experience, I would recommend that friends and family members of those with pancreatic cancer do everything they can to make every experience a positive one for the patient – and that means allowing the patient 100% of their life and treatment.

9. **LEGAL DOCUMENTS AND HOSPICE**:

    Please see discussion on these topics later in this book.

CHAPTER SEVEN

QUESTIONS FOR PRIMARY DOCTOR AND/OR ONCOLOGIST

The following is a list of questions to ask your primary care physician and/or oncologist once the possibility of pancreatic cancer is brought up.

1. **Do I have Pancreatic Cancer?**
   - How did you come to this conclusion?
   - What type of pancreatic Cancer do I have? Where is the tumor? What size is the tumor? Does the tumor extend beyond the pancreas? Has the tumor invaded any blood vessels or nerves? What are the margins of the tumor (is there normal tissue on all sides of it? Is it encased in fat?)
   - What stage is the pancreatic Cancer?
   - If my biopsy was negative, I would like to be referred to a medical oncologist who specializes in gastrointestinal cancer for follow-up and further testing.
   - Has my pancreatic Cancer metastasized? Where to? How much? How do you know it has metastasized?

2. **While we are waiting for the oncologist appointment, can you please prescribe a 3 Phase Pancreatic Protocol CT Scan with contrast which will assist the oncologist with staging and treatment decisions?**

3. Can I have referrals to the following healthcare providers:

   *Note: You may want just an initial referral to a good medical oncologist - and then ask the medical oncologist for referrals for the rest of the following healthcare team members.

   1. **Medical Oncologist (specializing in gastrointestinal cancers)**:
      This doctor will be the team leader and will assist with an overall treatment plan, including chemo.

   2. **Radiation Oncologist**:
      This doctor will evaluate you for radiation treatment.

   3. **Surgical Oncologist (specializing in gastrointestinal cancers)**:
      This doctor will evaluate you for surgery.

   4. **Palliative Care Doctor**:
      This doctor will assist with keeping you feeling good and ensuring you have a good quality of life.

   5. **Pain Specialist**:
      This doctor will ensure that you not only have medication for pain, but also medication for breakthrough pain when it occurs.

   6. **Nutritionist**:
      The nutritionist will help with weight maintenance and nutrition both before, during and after the treatment process.

7. **Social Worker**:

   The social worker can help with utilizing community resources to assist you with your treatment and end of life care such as counseling, free medical beds, free transportation, economic resources, home assistance, hospice, etc…

8. **Therapist**:

   A therapist can help patients and their families cope with the cancer diagnosis, treatment issues, depression (which is common in people with cancer), and with end of life issues.

9. **Hospice**:

   I recommend calling and visiting a hospice facility or group as soon as pancreatic cancer is diagnosed. Hospice assists with providing care and comfort for anyone with a terminal diagnosis who decides to stop treating their cancer. Medicare covered my dad's hospice 100%. The purpose of hospice is to enable a terminally ill person who no longer wants any treatment (or where having any more treatment would be futile) to live out their remaining time with as little discomfort as possible. The emphasis is on quality of life and comfort.

4. **Is my Pancreatic Cancer resectable? Why or why not?**
    - What stage is it? What does the staging category I'm in mean?
    - Is it locally advanced (wrapped around or near artery/vessels) or metastatic (spread to distant organs like liver or peritoneum)?
    - Is it possible, after receiving chemo and/or radiation, that if the cancer shrinks that I might become eligible for resection?
    - I want to have the Whipple Surgery at a center that performs 20 or more Whipple Surgeries per year, what hospital can you recommend that meets that requirement?

5. **What is my prognosis?**

    NOTE: You do not have to ask this and you can even tell the doctor that you do not want to know your prognosis. Also, if you ask this question, please note that many people have longer or shorter than 3-6 months, it all depends on the condition of your body, if you receive treatment, how your tumor responds to treatment, and luck. And remember, doctors do NOT have crystal balls and they can never with any accuracy tell you exactly how long you have to live. Doctors can only provide educated guesses based on your condition.

6. **What is your personal experience in treating patients with pancreatic cancer? How many patients in the past year?**

7. **What treatment do you recommend and why?**
    - What is the goal of treatment?
    - What are the risks of the treatment?
    - How will the treatment affect my quality of life?
    - How will you know if the treatment is working?
    - What is the next step if the initial treatment plan isn't working?
    - How will I feel during and after treatment?
    - What are the side effects to the treatments I will be receiving?
    - What do I need to do to care for myself during this treatment?
    - Will I be able to continue my usual activities during treatment?
    - For what reasons should I call your office during my treatment? (i.e., fever over a certain temperature, blood pressure under a certain number, vomiting or diarrhea exceeding a specific number of hours or days, etc...)?
    - What symptoms should cause me to go to the emergency room right away?
    - Can you prescribe an intravenous antiemetic to be provided along with the chemo?

8. **Before the first chemo can you prescribe (in liquid form if possible - easier to swallow):**
    1. Pain meds and Break through pain meds
    2. Anti-nausea meds and Anti-diarrheal meds and specifically anti-nausea meds I can take with my IV chemotherapy
    3. Anti-cramping meds
    4. Something to reduce risk of blood clots (low weight molecule heparin?)

5. Pulsing or Low Dose Antibiotic to Ward off Infections (especially with patients who have bile duct stents).

9. When should I start being concerned about ascites (fluid buildup in the abdomen)?

10. When should I start being concerned about pancreatic enzymes being insufficient or malnutrition from having a blocked pancreatic duct?

11. What vitamins/supplements might be helpful or harmful throughout this treatment?

12. Many people who get pancreatic cancer also can acquire diabetes (pancreatic issues) or also low blood sugar (due to chemo), what should I be doing to monitor for diabetes or blood sugar levels? Should I take a sugar pill if my blood sugar gets too low? What would be considered "low" blood sugar?

13. Should any of the following be done ahead of time while my body is stronger: bile duct bypass, nerve block or gallbladder removal?

14. What do I need to know with regard to my current medical conditions and medications will affect treatment and treatment options?

15. Jaundice, Bile Duct Stricture (narrowing) and Pancreatic Duct Stricture (narrowing):
    A lot of people who have pancreatic cancer eventually get jaundice (yellowing of the skin and eyes), can you explain what this means?
    - Do I have jaundice now?
    - Should I expect to eventually get jaundice?
    - What signs do I have to watch out for with regard to jaundice?
    - If I have it now, what will be done to correct it?
    - Will I be receiving a plastic stent, metal stent or coated metal stent in my bile duct and why?
    - ****If I receive a metal stent in my bile duct, will I be able to have the Whipple surgery later?
    - What are the symptoms of a stent dislodging and what should I do if that occurs?
    - How narrow is my bile duct and/or pancreatic duct?
    - What is acute pancreatitis and what causes it?
    - Should I change my eating habits to ward off acute pancreatitis?
    - Do I need to take pancreatic enzymes?

16. **Prepping for Chemo**:

   Can we start a weight gain program right now? Drinking ensure or boost - and eating high calorie food with high protein content?

CHAPTER EIGHT

UNDERSTANDING THE NUANCES OF PANCREATIC CANCER

Pancreatic cancer is THE most difficult cancer to diagnose and treat. Skin cancer can usually be spotted and removed since it occurs on the surface of the body. Breast cancer is often felt just under the skin and can be removed. Pancreatic cancer has some very unique properties that patients should familiarize themselves with.

1. **HARD TO VISUALIZE**:

    The pancreas is hidden behind the stomach and it can be difficult to visualize or feel the tumor(s) with traditional testing and examination techniques. Early pancreatic cancer cells closely resemble normal pancreas tissue which also makes it difficult to see early pancreatic cancer on various types of imaging tests.

2. **NO EARLY DETECTION**:

    There is no early detection screening available for pancreatic cancer. There is no urine or blood test to detect pancreatic cancer. Most blood and urine tests that have attempted at detecting pancreatic cancer in its early stages are foiled because pancreatic cancer and pancreatitis attacks (inflammation of the pancreas) tend to release similar chemicals, enzymes and proteins which make it difficult to distinguish whether someone has cancer or pancreatitis. Without early detection, pancreatic cancer has more time to spread which makes it even more difficult to remove it.

3. **ELDERLY POPULATION GETS IT MORE**:

   Pancreatic cancer tends to occur more often in elderly populations who usually have other health problems which may prevent treatment from being an option.

4. **OCCURS IN CENTRAL LOCATION OF BODY**:

   Pancreatic cancer occurs in an area of the body that is very central to a lot of systems the body needs to function. The fact that it appears in an area so close to many vital body systems makes it more likely to do harm faster and spread faster than other cancers.

5. **AFFECTS THE ENTIRE BODY**:

   Pancreatic cancer is not just a tumor, but also presents itself as a "syndrome" whereby it affects and weakens the entire body and its systems.

6. **METASTASIZES EARLY**:

   Pancreatic cancer cells tend to microscopically metastasize early in the course of the disease. The cells are excellent at sticking around somewhere in the body and will usually cause a reoccurrence of the cancer even if surgery is performed to remove the original tumor. The recurrence rate post surgery is about 85%! A laboratory mouse that had been given pancreatic cancer was found to shed microscopic pancreatic cancer cells throughout its body before a tumor even developed!

7. **SUPPRESSES IMMUNE SYSTEM**:

    Pancreatic cancer cells will suppress the local immune system to prevent the immune system from fighting it. The pancreatic cancer tumor forms a type of "shield" that prevents the body's immune fighting T cells from getting close to it.

8. **ENCAPSULATES SELF**:

    Pancreatic cancer tumors tend to encapsulate themselves in a hardened "shell" called stroma (a fibrous tissue), which makes it much more difficult for chemotherapy, radiation and other treatments to penetrate and get into the actual tumor itself. Newer studies show that the stroma may actually help prevent the cancer from spreading faster and it may be your body's way of helping to contain the cancer. Regardless, the stroma still makes effective chemotherapy and radiation treatment difficult.

9. **POOR PERFUSION**:

    Pancreatic tumors tend to have poor perfusion, meaning that they don't develop very much of a vascular system. What this means is that it is very difficult for IV chemotherapy to reach the tumor.

10. **NAKED ORGAN**:

    The Pancreas is one of the few internal organs without a membrane - which makes it easier for cancer cells to migrate elsewhere in the body.

11. **WRAPS ITSELF AROUND MAJOR VESSELS**:

    Pancreatic cancer tumors tend to wrap themselves around major blood vessels and nerves which run through the pancreas - which often makes surgical removal impossible and helps enable the cancer to metastasize faster.

12. **CAN MUTATE ITSELF AGAINST TREATMENTS**:

    Pancreatic cancer can rapidly alter itself so that if a treatment (i.e., chemo) is used, the cells can mutate to form a very quick resistance to that particular treatment. Scientists have recently learned that not all cancer cells are the same – they can differ from each other. A pancreatic cancer tumor can have one type of cell, it metastasizes elsewhere in the body and the new tumor in the lymph node can be a very different type of pancreatic cancer cell. The cancer cells in the pancreas tumor may be very susceptible to a type of chemo while a metastasized tumor is completely resistant to the tumor in the lymph node. Pancreatic cancer cells can mutate quite rapidly.

13. **CREATES AN ENVIRONMENT RESISTENT TO RADIATION AND CHEMOTHERAPY**:

    Pancreatic cancer tumors are very "hypoxic" - meaning that they create an environment for themselves that lack oxygen. Radiation therapy requires an environment with oxygen to be effective; therefore, radiation often will not work to eliminate pancreatic cancer tumors. Chemotherapy also does a better job of affecting cancerous tumors in more oxygen rich environments. Scientists have recently started to test out the effectiveness of injecting pancreatic tumors with oxygen rich molecules to aid chemotherapy and radiation with killing the tumor.

14. **TUMOR VISUALIZATION**:

If the tumor can be visualized on a scan, then the tumor picture is often blurry with undefined borders. This makes it difficult to accurately determine staging and to determine if it is the tumor is resectable (able to be removed) or not.

15. **CA19-9**:

In some people (about 70%) who have been diagnosed with pancreatic cancer, there is a blood tumor marker (CA19-9) that goes up and down depending on the size of the tumor. It is an unreliable early cancer screening detection test. It only helps, along with other factors, to discover whether treatment for the cancer is effective.

16. **BLOOD CLOTS**:

Pancreatic cancer is known to increase the risk of blood clots. Doctors can prescribe medications to help prevent blood clots from occurring. Doctors can also educate patients on how to identify a possible blood clot so that the patient can get himself to the emergency room right away for treatment.

17. **JAUNDICE**:

If the first symptom of your pancreatic cancer is painless jaundice, then it is much more likely that your tumor will qualify for surgical removal with the Whipple Surgery than if the cancer presents itself in other ways (i.e., pain, weight loss and gastrointestinal discomfort).

CHAPTER NINE
PERFORMANCE STATUS

One of the determining factors as to what treatment a pancreatic cancer patient can qualify for is known as the Performance Status of an individual. Performance Status provides a way to determine the overall general health of a patient in order to help determine what treatments they qualify for.

It's recommended that pancreatic cancer patients find out Performance Status so that appropriate treatment options can be selected. *For example, based on my own father's Performance Status, it would have been completely unreasonable for him to have been given chemotherapy. My father, had a sizable aortic aneurysm, a pacemaker for his heart, had several heart stents with some occluded, had high blood pressure, was 85 years old, had significant arthritis, was on blood thinners, etc... He ultimately was not a good candidate for any pancreatic cancer treatment due to his overall health status. Up until his jaundice, he lived independently and could care for himself, but his overall health was not very good.*

The Performance Status scale was developed by the Eastern Cooperative Oncology Group (ECOG) in 1982. The scale is as follows:

Grade	ECOG Performance Status
0	Fully active, able to carry on all pre-disease performance without restriction
1	Restricted in physically strenuous activity but ambulatory and able to carry out work of a light or sedentary nature (i.e., light house work or office work)
2	Ambulatory and capable of all selfcare but unable to carry out any work activities; up and about more than 50% of waking hours
3	Capable of only limited selfcare; confined to bed or chair more than 50% of waking hours
4	Completely disabled, cannot carry on any selfcare; totally confined to bed or chair
5	Deceased

The other scale used to assess the functional status of a patient is the Karnofsky Performance Status

Grade	Karnofsky Performance Status
100	Normal, no complaints; no evidence of disease
90	Able to carry on normal activity; minor signs or symptoms of disease
80	Normal activity with effort, some signs or symptoms of disease
70	Cares for self but unable to carry on normal activity or to do active work
60	Requires occasional assistance but is able to care for most of personal needs
50	Requires considerable assistance and frequent medical care
40	Disabled, requires special care and assistance
30	Severely disabled, hospitalization is indicated although death is not imminent
20	Very ill; hospitalization and active support care necessary
10	Moribund
0	Deceased

Comparing the ECOG Performance Status with Karnofsky Performance Status

ECOG		**Karnofsky**
0	=	100 or 90
1	=	80 or 70
2	=	60 or 50
3	=	40 or 30
2	=	20 or 10
0	=	0

CHAPTER TEN

PANCREATIC CANCER TREATMENT OPTIONS

1. **SURGERY** :

    * Pancreatic cancer can be difficult to see in scans. If Pancreatic cancer appears to be resectable (i.e., removable via surgery), then Whipple Surgery or a variation of the Whipple Surgery is used to remove the tumor.

    * Surgery is the only known possible "cure" for pancreatic cancer, but in most cases the cancer eventually comes back (85% recurrence rate) even when surgery is performed (most often it recurs in the liver).

    * The surgery is a long surgery (8-10 hours) with a very difficult and long recovery period.

    * The surgery is worth the effort with a chance to extend life by a number of years and a chance to possibly cure the cancer itself.

    * If Whipple Surgery is attempted and the surgeon discovers that the tumor is inoperable or the cancer has spread, the surgeon may perform a smaller surgery to prevent symptoms (i.e., a bile duct blockage) or abort the surgery all together. About 30% of those who qualify for surgery will have the surgery aborted on the operating table due to a finding of ascites (fluids accumulating in abdomen which indicate death is near), finding the tumor has metastasized or finding the tumor has enveloped major body structures and cannot be removed safely.

* If the tumor is deemed to be **Borderline Resectable**, then chemo and radiation treatment must be used in an attempt to shrink the tumor so that it becomes surgically resectable.

2. **CHEMOTHERAPY**:

   * Usually not curative unless it gets helps make a borderline resectable tumor shrink down enough to become resectable.

   * Treatment time varies

   * It is most commonly used to slow the progression of the cancer, increase quality of life and reduce pain

   * May also be used after the Whipple Surgery in an attempt to kill any remaining cancer cells floating around in the body

   * With pancreatic cancer, it is common for chemotherapy to fail to shrink the tumor. If it does shrink the tumor, the cancer will often adapt (become resistant) so that eventually the chemotherapy regimen being used is no longer effective. This means that that a different type of chemo will need to be used from that point forward. In addition, cancer cells can have different genetic codes (just like some people can have brown hair, blonde hair or red hair). If you have different types of pancreatic cancer cells, then chemotherapy may only be successful in

attacking one specific type while the other types of pancreatic cancer cells proliferate.

* **Chemotherapy Drugs Currently Used:**

  1. **GEMCITABINE along with Abraxane, Tarceva and/or Xeloda:**
     * Usually not as "harsh" as FolFirinox Treatment
     * An average life extension of 6.8 months
     * In a well known French study, about 9% of patients had some tumor shrinkage

  2. **FOLFIRINOX (consists of a combination of Flourouracil (5-FU), Irinotecan Hydrochloride, Leucovorin Calcium and Oxaliplatin):**
     * For healthier people who can handle the harder side effects, and with an average life extension of 11.1 months
     * To qualify for it, usually need a performance status of a 1 or 2, be younger than 76 and have good liver function
     * A higher risk for people who have biliary stents because there is a higher risk for neutropenia. Neutropenia puts people with stents at higher risk for infections that can lead to sepsis (fatal blood infection)
     * In the well known French study on FolFirinox, about 1/3 of the patients had some tumor shrinkage

- Ask for EMEND to be added to chemotherapy IV for antinausea.

- **Experimental Chemotherapy**: Pancreatic cancer is not as susceptible to chemotherapy as other cancer types due to its special physical characteristics (hypoxic environment, encapsulation, etc…). Some doctors are experimenting with directly injecting the tumor with chemotherapy to get around those characteristics.

3. **RADIATION**:
    - Low dose radiation therapy targeting liver and pancreas.
    - 3D Conformal Radiation Therapy - Pancreas
    - **CyberKnife**:

    Radiation therapy that actually accounts for your respiratory movements and the radiation beam will "follow" the tumor around as your breathe - less chance of affecting healthy tissue surrounding tumor.
    - **Experimental Radiation Therapy**:

    Pancreatic cancer tumors are hypoxic tumors – meaning that the tumor creates a low oxygen environment. Radiation treatment works best if the area being treated is oxygen rich. Some doctors are experimenting with injecting oxygenated cells into pancreatic cancer tumors to make them more susceptible to radiation therapy.

4. **BIOLOGIC MEDICATIONS**:
   - Use in combination with chemotherapy
   - Some used are: Herceptin and Erbitux

5. **TARGETED THERAPY**:
   1. **Experimental Drugs - Targeting The Ras Gene**:
      Pancreatic cancer has mutations in ras gene and malignant cells contain the unique enzyme (farnesyl transferase). The drugs being developed try to target this enzyme and are currently in clinical trials. These drugs include Tarceva, Sutent and Afinitor.

   2. **Experimental Vaccines**:
      GVAX or Virulizin are two different pancreatic cancer vaccines that are currently undergoing clinical trials.

6. **EXPERIMENTAL PHOTO DYNAMIC THERAPY**:
   Photo Dynamic Therapy causes local necrosis of tissue with light after the prior administration of a photosensitizing drug (Meso-tetrahdroxyphenyl Chlorine via IV).

7. **EXPERIMENTAL VITAMINS AND SUPPLEMENTS**:
   A Specialized Vitamin D was being studied in 2014 for possible treatment of pancreatic cancer.

8. **CLINICAL TRIALS**:

The rate of pancreatic cancer and the length of life after diagnosis has not changed much over 40 years. Currently, there is a push to try to cure or lengthen the life span of people with pancreatic cancer. Since the prognosis is so dismal, many pancreatic cancer patients ask their oncologists for information on clinical trials. There are many ongoing clinical trials for new drugs, new therapies or new drug therapy combinations for pancreatic cancer patients. For many pancreatic cancer patients, participating in a clinical trial can give them hope that a trial treatment will cure them, lengthen their life span or give them a sense of peace that their participation could possibly prevent others from having to suffer with such a deadly disease. Information about available drug trials can be found online through various pancreatic cancer organizations, at university hospitals, at cancer centers and from your oncologist.

CHAPTER ELEVEN

RESEARCH INTO PANCREATIC CANCER TREATMENTS

Worldwide, different teams of scientists are working on earlier treatment detection of and on a cure for pancreatic Cancer. Following are just some of the latest discoveries (as of 2016):

Earlier Detection:
Scientists are working on blood tests and urine tests to find pancreatic cancer earlier. The theory is that, like other cancers, the cure rate for pancreatic cancer may increase dramatically if the cancer is detected at its earliest stages. Scientists are focusing on detecting early migrating metastasized pancreatic cancer cells in human blood. They are also trying to identify special pancreatic cancer-related proteins in the blood and urine so that earlier detection may be possible.

Recently, a US doctor started using a WATS-3D platform which gives a high-definition view of samples from the pancreas. The hope is to eventually customize treatment based upon a patient's particular type of pancreatic cancer cells. There are also other tools that are being used to experiment with to scan the wall of the pancreas and destroy cancerous cells.

Personalized Cancer Treatment:

Some scientists are working on ways to customize treatment for pancreatic cancer based on both a patient's stroma and tumor subtype. Researchers have found that there are different subtypes of pancreatic cancer tumors, a "basal-like" tumor that is associated with a poorer prognosis and a "classical" subtype which was a bit of a better prognosis for surviving to a year. Customizing medicine based on stroma and tumor subtype may improve the effectiveness of treatments.

Electricity and Tumor Treatment:

Electroporation uses electrical fields to burn holes in cell membranes which kills the cells. The use of "irreversible electroporation (IRE) doubles the survival time for patients with locally advanced pancreatic cancer, according to research published in the *Annals of Surgery* (2015; doi:10.1097/SLA.0000000000001441)." The "appropriate and precise use of IRE in appropriately selected patients with locally advanced pancreatic cancer can result in a median overall survival close to 24 months, which is nearly double the survival rate with the best new chemotherapy and chemoradiotherapy," said first author Robert C.G. Martin, II, MD, PhD, director of surgical oncology at the University of Louisville in Kentucky.

Drug Research:

Drug research recently revealed that two drugs, JQ1 and Vorinostat, shrank pancreatic cancer tumors in lab mice by chemically modifying the cancer's DNA (epigenetic therapy). Most cases of pancreatic cancer are linked to the gene

KRAS which makes a protein that helps to control how cells grow. Epigenetic science is trying to use these new experimental drugs to interfere with cancer cell reproduction.

The anti-diabetic drug, Metformin, has been shown to possibly increase the life span of those with pancreatic cancer. Most cancers rely on glycolysis (sugar energy) to grow, but pancreatic cancer relies on oxygen to grow. Metformin might interfere with the cancer's energy supply.

Clinical studies are currently underway with the drug Nab-paclitaxel along with the classic pancreatic cancer chemotherapy drug, gemcitabine. When the two drugs were combined, they appear to extend the lifespan of those who had a failed response to Folfirinox chemotherapy treatment.

Vaccine for Pancreatic Cancer:
Lei Zheng, MD, PhD, and his colleagues at the Johns Hopkins Kimmel Cancer Center in Baltimore, Maryland, have shown a relationship between annexin A2 and Sema3D in patients with pancreatic cancer. Annexin A2 draws Sema3D out of the pancreatic cancer cells and aids somehow in the spread of the cancer. The goal is to develop a vaccine that targets annexin A2 and a small molecule to inhibit Sema3D with the hope of halting the metastasis of pancreatic cancer.

Immunotherapy:

Doctors at MD Anderson Cancer Center recently discovered that the stroma in pancreatic cancer tumors are extremely thick compared to other cancers. It has long been thought that if the stroma could be gotten rid of then the cancer could be attacked more easily with chemotherapy. In studies, the MD Anderson doctors found that the opposite was true! The destruction of the stroma actually made the cancer grow faster! The doctors found that tumors with smaller amounts of stroma "emitted a special chemical to weaken the immune system, and when this chemical was blocked it helped to lengthen the life of mice." Scientists are studying how the human immune system responds to pancreatic cancer and using this new information to formulate treatments in a new science called immunotherapy. A top immunologist in the US who won the Nobel Prize was stricken with pancreatic cancer. He attempted to kill his cancer cells by trying to teach a particular immune cell, called a drendite, to attack and kill the cancer cells. He died before being able to perfect the technique.

CHAPTER TWELVE

SYMPTOMS OF PANCREATIC CANCER AND SIDE EFFECTS OF CANCER TREATMENTS

When people think of cancer, they often think "tumor"; however, pancreatic cancer is a WHOLE BODY illness. The entire body's chemistry system changes due to the existence of cancer. These changes in body chemistry make the body more susceptible to various infections and medical conditions.

Many cancer related symptoms overlap with treatment symptoms. It is suggested that each patient keep a daily "health journal" to keep record of every health problem encountered so that it will be easier for doctors to identify causes and treat them more effectively. With pancreatic cancer patients, it is also helpful to keep track of food and beverage intake.

The following list is not an all-inclusive list of possible side effects or symptoms, but I did try to include most of them. Not all of the following symptoms or side effects will occur to every patient; however, becoming familiar with them can help patients be better prepared for their journey.

1. **DEEP VEIN THROMBOSIS (DVT) & BLOOD CLOTS**

    Pancreatic cancer causes changes in the blood that can increase the likelihood of forming blood clots in the veins (usually veins of the legs). This condition, known as Deep Vein Thrombosis (DVT), usually causes symptoms like swelling, pain or tenderness. Pay particular attention if swelling occurs in just one leg. Notify a doctor right away if you DVT is suspected.

It is possible for a DVT blood clot to break loose (an embolus) and travel to the lungs (pulmonary embolism), head (stroke) or heart (heart attack). Wear loose fitted clothing and do not wear tight shoes, socks or pants. Ask the doctor about wearing compression stockings.

Treatment consists of anticoagulant drugs that thin the blood, prevent existing clots from increasing in size and prevent new clots from forming. Ask the doctor about Low Molecular Weight Heparin (LMWH). Since cancer makes the body more prone to clotting, ask your doctor if, based on your personal health history, you should start taking an anticoagulant before DVT develops. Keep in mind that anti-coagulants thin the blood. Some anti-coagulants can be medically "deactivated" right away with counteracting medications while other coagulants cannot be medically "deactivated" which can cause surgical delays.

2. **PAIN**:

    Pancreatic cancer usually will cause pain at some point in the disease process (usually in the abdominal area, but also may be experienced in the back or other areas). The pain is caused by the tumor invading organs and nerves – or by causing narrowing, blockages, pressure and interfering with body systems. This interference will cause inflammation or fluid backing up in places where it should not be. It is important to ask your doctor for a referral to a palliative care specialist or a pain specialist as soon as you are diagnosed with pancreatic cancer so that you can be prepared for the pain if it occurs.

    My father was very concerned about "becoming addicted" to narcotics when I or others gently encouraged him to ask the doctor about getting a prescription for pain medication. We are all taught that becoming addicted to narcotics is a terrible thing. The truth is, when someone uses narcotics to treat actual pain - their chance of becoming addicted is extremely low. When someone who is not in pain decides to abuse narcotics, the narcotic changes the brain chemistry to create addiction.

    Also, those with pancreatic cancer generally have such a short amount of life left, that the last thing that they should worry about is an addiction to narcotics. No one has to or needs to live with any amount of pain - especially when it comes to pancreatic cancer. In addition, treating the pain associated with pancreatic cancer can help improve the quality of life and may even extend it a bit longer because stress caused by pain can interfere with treatments and general overall health.

When we have a headache, we usually take a pill and the headache goes away. When it comes to cancer and pain, there is a different method of treating pain.

A baseline dosage of an opioid is usually prescribed for the constant abdominal pain that may be experienced by those with pancreatic cancer. In addition to the "normal" amount of pain prevention, a patient may also experience what is called "break-through pain". "Break-through pain" is a short period of time where the pain gets to such a high level that the normal opioid prescribed is not adequate to control the pain. To combat this issue, a doctor will usually also prescribe a **"break-through pain" medication** to take in addition to the opioid when "break-through pain" occurs. If a patient experiences enough episodes of "break-through pain", then the doctor will usually increase the baseline dosage of the opioid. It is important to keep a record of your "break-through pain" episodes, and ask the doctor to increase the baseline opioid dosage if you find yourself constantly needing the "break-through pain" medication to control pain.

It is common for pancreatic cancer tumors to invade the nerve bundles in the back. A Celiac Plexus Neurolysis (CPD) is a nerve block available to eliminate this type of pain. You can get this in advance to reduce dependence on opioids. This treatment involves a doctor injecting alcohol into the nerve bundle which is frequently affected by pancreatic cancer tumors. Radiation therapy may also be effective in reducing pain when the tumor has grown into the Celiac Plexus.

Pain medications have side effects which include sleepiness, nausea and constipation. Sleepiness usually passes, but doctors can prescribe stool softners and laxatives to take with pain medication. If pain medications cause dizziness or confusion, notify the doctor so that he can prescribe a different dosage or a different medication that is better tolerated. Over time, patients using pain medications may find that their pain medication has become less effective. Pain medication dosages can always be increased by a doctor to conquer any amount of pain, so do not live with the pain and make sure to notify your doctor the current dosage is no longer effective. You can also request a referral to a pain specialist for more intense management.

There are options when it comes to pain medications. A lot of people who get pancreatic cancer are elderly and have difficulty swallowing. Pain medications are available as patches, suckers, intravenous pump and suppositories. Let your doctor know if you have trouble swallowing and need a different route for your medication.

3. **BILARY STRICTURE (NARROWING OF THE BILE DUCT)**
Often, the pancreatic cancer tumor will put pressure on the bile duct and cause it to narrow or become blocked. If the bile duct is narrowed or blocked, then this can stop bile from flowing freely into the intestines to aid in digestion.

This blockage of bile will cause jaundice to occur. Jaundice is the name of the condition where the eyes and skin turn a yellowish hue. Symptoms that accompany jaundice usually include pale colored stools, dark urine and itchy skin. (My dad had painless jaundice without itchiness).

Biliary stricture can be fixed with:
- Surgical insertion of a metal stent (if Whipple surgery isn't a possibility)
- Surgical insertion of a plastic stent (which does not last as long as a metal stent, but which will keep the option of having the Whipple surgery)
- Surgical bile bypass where the bile duct is bypassed and the bile flows outside of the body into an outside pouch

NOTE: SEE THE NEXT CHAPTER ON STENTS

If the stent is dislodged, fails or the bile duct becomes strictured elsewhere, then the jaundice can recur. In this case, the stent will need to be replaced or bile bypass surgery will need to be performed.

4. **INFECTIONS AND LOW WHITE BLOOD CELL COUNT:**

People who have pancreatic cancer are more prone to infections. Poor nutrition, diminished function of the liver, pancreas and other organs, immobility and suppression of the immune system by both the cancer and treatments for cancer (chemo) lowers resistance to infections. Patients with biliary stents are more prone to infections than those without stents.

Symptoms of infection can include pain, fever of 100.5 F and higher, shaking, chills, sore throat or cough, increased frequency or burning while urinating, swelling, redness, pain anywhere on skin, vomiting or diarrhea and rapid breathing.

Infections are routinely treated with antibiotics (oral or IV infused). For patients who are receiving chemotherapy treatment, if white blood cell counts drops too low, the doctor may be able to prescribe Neopogen or Neulasta. Patients who have internal stents are more prone to infection, so it may be useful to ask the doctor for a pulsing or low dose antibiotic therapy to help ward off cholangitis (infected bile duct) and other types of infections.

Infections can partially be prevented by washing the hands (bathroom, before and after eating, after going out in public), taking daily baths or showers, brushing teeth daily, avoiding the sharing of food utensils and beverages, and avoiding people who are sick. Make sure to check with the doctor before having dental work or receiving immunizations of any kind.

5. **MALDIGESTION**:

Maldigestion is the body's inability to properly digest what you eat or drink. Maldigestion is very different from having a poor appetite or indigestion. Maldigestion occurs internally AFTER food/drink are consumed. The amount ingested has no bearing on maldigestion. Most maldigestion is associated with the pancreatic tumor either pressing on or invading the pancreatic and bile ducts causing a total or partial blockage of those ducts.

Many people with pancreatic cancer will suffer from maldigestion because the amount of pancreatic enzymes available to aid in digestion are decreased (pancreatic Exocrine Insufficiency (PEI)) due to a narrowed or blocked pancreatic duct. Those with pancreatic cancer can also suffer maldigestion because bile, a product of the liver which aids in digestion, is unable to reach the intestines due to a blocked or partially blocked bile duct. A partially or completely blocked duodenum (small intestines) due to tumor growth may also prevent normal digestion.

In addition to surgical options explained in the next chapter, doctors can prescribe medication known as pancreatic Lipase. Pancreatic Lipase is taken orally along with food and helps replace some of the pancreatic enzymes that you may not be getting internally. A typical dosage is 40,000 - 70,000 IU with meals and 20,000-25,000 IU with snacks; however, a doctor may need to adjust the dosage to each patient's needs.

Patients may also want to ask their doctor for medication to suppress gastric acid. These medications are referred to as H2 Blockers or Proton-

Pump Inhibitors. These medications prevent the inactivation of enzymes and improve the efficacy of enzymes.

6. **BOWEL OBSTRUCTION**:

    The pancreatic cancer tumor can grow into the upper part of the small intestines (aka duodenum) and cause a blockage in digestion either by putting pressure on the intestines or by growing into the intestines. Bowel obstruction can also be caused by compaction of fecal matter due to constipation (often from pain medicines). Bowel obstruction can also be caused by what are called surgical adhesions (scar tissue that forms after a surgical procedure in the intestines or radiation treatment in the abdominal area). Finally, bowel obstruction can be caused by tumors that grow into the nerves affecting bowel function.

    The symptoms of bowel obstruction include:
    - Crampy and intermittent abdominal pain with or without vomiting
    - Pain that lasts for several days and gets worse over time accompanied by abdominal distention (swollen belly)
    - Nausea
    - Diarrhea
    - Constipation - No Bowel Movements or Flatulence (Gas)
    - Fever
    - Tachycardia (Increased heart rate)

    Various medications can be provided to increase comfort like analgesics for pain, subcutaneous fluids (hydration fluids injected under the skin), antiemetics for vomiting, steroids for inflammation, a "prokinetic agent" (metoclopramide) that helps "move stuff along" and can assist with partial obstructions, medication for spasms and nausea (hyoscine butylbromide), medication to reduce pressure within the bowel (Octreotide) and a medication that is stronger than laxatives (Amidotrizoate).

7. **ACUTE PANCREATITIS ATTACK:**

An acute pancreatitis attack is an inflammation of Pancreas due to pancreatic juices backing up into the Pancreas. The reason pancreatic juices cannot drain out of the pancreas adequately is because the pancreatic duct is narrowed or blocked due to pressure or in-growth of the pancreatic cancer tumor.

Normally, pancreatic juices are not activated until they enter into the small intestines. If their passage is blocked and they cannot enter into the small intestines, then they will "activate" inside the pancreas itself! Essentially, these pancreatic juices will start digesting the pancreas! In reaction to this, the pancreas will become very inflamed and infected (acute pancreatitis).

Acute pancreatitis can cause sepsis, organ failure and death. Severe acute pancreatitis has a high mortality rate (approximately 25%).

Acute pancreatitis is a hospital emergency and the symptoms include pain in the upper abdomen, chest or back, nausea and vomiting, diarrhea, fever, rapid pulse or slow pulse and possibly shortness of breath.

Normal Treatment of Pancreatitis:

Includes a visit to the hospital to acquire IV Fluids (so the pancreas can rest), no oral nutrition for 24-48 hours to rest the pancreas, narcotic pain medications for pain, medications for nausea, medications for infection and possibly surgical insertion of a catheter for the pancreatic duct to help the pancreas heal. In some cases, the doctor may be able to use ERCP insert a stent or perform a balloon dilation on the pancreatic duct to keep it open. A main side effect of ERCP is pancreatitis, but sometimes it is needed.

Pancreatitis Treatment with Pancreatic Cancer Patients:

Acute pancreatitis can be partially prevented by eating frequent smaller meals instead of three large regular meals per day. Also, eating a low fat diet and limiting alcohol consumption can help.

If a pancreatic cancer patient continually gets acute pancreatitis, a surgical intervention may be necessary.

Unfortunately, my father had two attacks of acute pancreatitis right before his death. I do not believe the doctors adequately counseled him on how he should be eating due to his narrowed pancreatic duct. I believe that these back-to-back incidences of acute pancreatitis hastened his death. **NOTE: If you have any narrowing of the pancreatic duct, please do everything you can to eat small frequent meals and ensure that you follow up with your doctor to do everything you can to prevent acute pancreatitis. Also, if you qualify for chemo and/or radiation therapy or the Whipple surgery, having an attack of acute pancreatitis can set you back a couple of weeks in your**

treatment - so it is best to do everything you can in your power to avoid any episodes of acute pancreatitis.

Pancreatic cancer patients also may want to insist on receiving Tramadol instead of morphine for pain associated with their cancer or acute pancreatitis. Morphine can increase biliary duct pressure and Tramadol does not appear to increase biliary duct pressure. For pancreatic cancer patients, this increase in biliary duct pressure can make a difference between whether their biliary duct becomes blocked or not.

In addition, when being treated for pancreatitis, pancreatic cancer patients may want to insist on receiving enteral nutrition (through a tube in the throat) as opposed to parenteral nutrition (through an IV drip). The reasoning is that when an IV drip is used, the gastrointestinal system is being bypassed. As a result, bacteria have a chance to flourish within the gastrointestinal system and cause sepsis and organ failure. With enteral nutrition, the gastrointestinal system is kept "busy" and bacteria do not have an opportunity to flourish or migrate. Enteral nutrition may help to prevent sepsis and organ failure. Enteral nutrition should be introduced within 24 hours of hospitalization and a tube down the nose can be used so that the patient can still talk. Pancreatic cancer patients are much more susceptible to infections in the gastrointestinal track and this method of treating pancreatitis may be more beneficial than the traditional approach.

8. **CANCER ASSOCIATED ANOREXIA-CACHEXIA SYNDROME (CACS) and GENERAL LOSS OF APPETITE:**

Pancreatic cancer changes chemical structures in the body which results in patients eating less, losing weight and losing muscle mass. The cancer itself can increase catabolic rate and systemic inflammation. The cancer also causes the body to need MORE calories than normal. The cancer usually results in altered taste perception, weakness, fullness, nausea, loss of appetite and marked protein wasting. Despite all of this, it is important for those suffering with pancreatic cancer who are eligible for chemotherapy, radiation and/or surgery to maintain their weight (and maybe even increase their weight if possible).

Your doctor may refer you to a nutritionist or he may recommend that you eat high-calorie high-protein foods and supplements (eggs, cottage cheese, yogurt, peanut butter on crackers, sandwiches with turkey or tuna, baked or broiled chicken, fish, beef, soups). You can also add butter, honey, jelly, sour cream, cheese, yogurt and cream to whatever it is you are eating. Limit what you drink WITH meals and try to drink in between meals instead (liquids will fill you up quicker before you have had a chance to eat the higher calorie meals). Limit caffeine and carbonated beverages which affect appetite. Rinse your mouth before eating to enhance the taste of food. Avoid eating alone if possible because we tend to eat more when we eat with others. We also tend to eat more when we eat while watching television or a movie.

Ask your doctor if you can take a nutritional supplement like Carnation Instant Breakfast, Ensure or Boost. Ask your doctor if you can have an alcoholic drink before you eat which can stimulate the appetite of some people. Doctors can prescribe Megestrol Acetate to improve appetite (although there is an increased risk of thrombosis (blood clots) with it). Doctors may be able to prescribe Thalidomide, Remeron, Marinol, Zyprexa, Olanzapine or other medications to also help with appetite.

It is important to follow your doctor's specific instructions because if your pancreatic duct is narrowed, then eating large meals may cause acute pancreatitis (which can delay treatments and may cause death).

My dad was not eating very much and he told me that he had been given Ensure in the hospital. He didn't like the flavor very much. I went to the store and got him both Ensure and Boost. The day before he went in for his last hospitalization, he tried the Boost and really enjoyed it. He felt that he probably would have liked the Ensure as well, but in the hospital they had given him the Ensure at room temperature instead of refrigerating it. Talk to your doctor before altering your diet in any way.

It's vital that family members not pressure those with pancreatic cancer into eating. They have enough stress to deal with and having family badgering them about eating can cause even more stress (which results in poorer health). Always allow the cancer patient to take the lead in their own care. If you are worried, gently ask them ONCE or TWICE to speak to their doctor about options to increase their appetite.

When Not to Worry About Food Intake:

Also, most people associate food with health, but when a patient's body is preparing itself to die, the gastrointestinal system is the first part of the body that is affected. This means that a patient will eat a lot less food than they normally would in the month or so preceding their death. It may be difficult, but when a cancer patient is suffering from end-stage cancer, family members need to be respectful of the process and not try to guilt the cancer patient into eating or try to force food on the cancer patient. Doing so can cause a more uncomfortable death for your loved one.

9. **DEPRESSION:**

Obviously, a cancer diagnosis can cause depression in anyone. Pancreatic cancer is a particularly deadly cancer and most patients quickly become aware of this. Despite this, it is important for those who are depressed or who think they might be depressed to get treatment for it by way of therapy and medication. Depression creates its own chemical stressors on the body and can amplify the ill effects of the cancer. Even if you are not clinically depressed, it really helps to talk to a therapist about being diagnosed, the ups and downs of treatment and facing end of life.

With treatment for depression, the body will be better able to withstand cancer treatments and also improve quality of life. Typical medications that can be used include Cymbalta or Effexor (for depression and pain) and Mirtzapine (for depression, insomnia and chemo induced nausea).

10. **ASCITES**:
Pronounced Ah-SITE-ees. When ascites is caused by cancer, it is known as "Malignant Ascites". Ascites is simply the build-up of fluid in the abdomen. About 20% of those with pancreatic cancer will get ascites and having ascites is usually a symptom that the patient is in the end stage of pancreatic cancer. Once ascites sets in, death is likely to come within a number of weeks and almost all medical professionals will recommend halting aggressive treatment to fight the cancer. If ascites is found during a Whipple surgery, surgeons will generally abort the surgery. The focus from that point on tends to be entirely on patient comfort.

Ascites can be caused by the following:
1. The cancer spreads to the abdominal lining, irritates the lining, and the lining produces fluids which build up in the abdomen.

2. The cancer spreads to the liver or portal vein which increases blood pressure and affects circulation resulting in fluid building up in the stomach.

3. The cancer affects the lymph system which cannot drain properly and lymph fluids are drained into the abdomen.

4. The cancer damages the liver which affects the production of blood protein and the body's circulation (ultimately resulting in fluid build-up in the abdomen).

5. The tumor itself may produce fluid that drains into the abdomen.

The symptoms of ascites include:
- Abdominal swelling, discomfort, audible fluid slushing around abdomen, increased waist circumference
- Sense of fullness and decreased appetite
- Nausea and/or vomiting
- Fatigue
- Ankle swelling
- Constipation
- Feeling of abdominal pain or pressure
- Indigestion
- Shortness of breath

Doctors usually attempt to control ascites by prescribing diuretics to help the body to eliminate excessive water and salt. Reducing your salt and liquid intake may be recommended. For a minority of people, taking diuretics can cause insomnia, skin problems, fatigue and low blood pressure. Taking diuretics does not always work and surgical options (like drainage), as described in the next chapter, are often used to provide temporary relief from ascites.

11. **CHOLANGITIS (BILE DUCT) INFECTION:**
Cholangitis is a life threatening infection of the bile duct which causes inflammation of the bile duct. It is an emergency condition that can be caused by a bacterial infection, blockage of the bile duct due to a gallstone,

stricture or failed stent (which allows bacteria to flourish), or by a tumor that has grown into or affected the bile duct. Having a stent in the bile duct or having previous bile duct surgery can make a patient more prone to getting cholangitis.

Symptoms include pain in the upper right side or upper middle part of the abdomen (or in the back right below the shoulder blade), fever, chills, shaking, dark urine and clay colored stools, nausea, vomiting, jaundice (yellowing of the skin and eyes), low blood pressure and confusion. "Reynolds' Pentad" is a combination of abdominal pain, jaundice, fever, septic shock and mental confusion - and usually indicates that the condition is getting worse and that sepsis (infection of the blood) is occurring. Elderly people may succumb to sepsis without the usual Reynolds' Pentad and those with a biliary stent may develop cholangitis without jaundice.

Cholangitis is usually treated with antibiotics and, if needed, a surgical procedure to remove the bile duct blockage. See the next chapter for surgical information.

12. **GALLBLADDER ATTACK:**

If the bile duct is blocked, the bile can accumulate in the gallbladder and cause an increase in pressure that can lead to rupture. Symptoms include abdominal tenderness and sudden pain in upper right abdomen that may gravitate toward the center of the belly or upper back and movement does not make the pain worse. Symptoms may also include gas, nausea, pain and discomfort after meals.

Treatment is to surgically unblock bile duct with stents and/or gallstone removal and surgical removal of gallbladder.

It is important to note that jaundice (turning yellow due to a bile duct blockage) is often caused by a gallstone making its way out of the gallbladder and into the bile duct. A gallstone blockage usually causes pain along with jaundice because the bile duct is trying to eliminate a stone by contracting and larger stones also tend to scrape the inside of the bile duct as they are being squeezed down the duct. With pancreatic cancer, many people have what is termed as "painless jaundice". My father was diagnosed with painless jaundice and they found a gallstone was stuck in his bile duct because the bile duct was severely narrowed due to the pancreatic tumor pressing on it. The bile duct was not contracting because it was narrowed from the tumor pressing on it. That's why he did not have pain with his jaundice.

13. **FATIGUE:**

The tumor can affect absorption of food by blocking or partially blocking the bile duct, pancreatic duct or small intestines. This results in malnutrition and anemia which can cause fatigue. Medications, surgeries, chemo, radiation and other treatments can also contribute to fatigue. A decrease in food intake, liquid intake, stress and pain can also contribute to fatigue. The cancer itself can reduce the number of red blood cells in the bloodstream and can cause anemia.

Symptoms of fatigue include feeling tired, weak, weary, lacking energy, inability to concentrate, and feeling irritable or depressed.

Fatigue can be addressed by surgically fixing the cause of malnutrition by consulting with a nutritionist. The doctor may be able to alter your medications. Try to sleep longer and take naps as needed. In addition, try to stay active and not lay in bed all day because laying in bed all day will decrease your overall energy level. Finally, learn to regulate your energy levels. If you have something important coming up, then rest before going to that activity. For example, my father was very weak and fatigued, but he wanted to take a shower in order to be clean for a doctor's appointment the next day. I encouraged him to take a full nap before he showered. After his nap, he had built up enough energy to complete his shower.

14. **INSOMNIA:**

Insomnia, or the inability to fall asleep or sleep peacefully can be caused by the cancer changing your metabolism, medications or general stress and anxiety. To remedy insomnia, try to keep to a regular sleep schedule and keep your daily nap to no more than one hour. Use relaxation techniques to help you get prepared to sleep. Ask the doctor to prescribe anti-anxiety medications if necessary.

15. **NAUSEA AND VOMITING**:

Both pancreatic Cancer and pancreatic Cancer treatment can cause nausea and vomiting. It is important to consult with your doctor so that he can figure out whether it is the treatment or the cancer causing the vomiting and then prescribe the right treatment. It is common for chemotherapy to be administered simultaneously with anti-nausea medication. Ask your doctor if he can prescribe chemotherapy along with the anti-nausea medication. Your doctor may also have you take anti-nausea medication just prior to your chemotherapy sessions. For people who have nausea and vomiting associated with the tumor or acute pancreatitis, the doctor may prescribe other types of medication or refer you to a nutritionist.

Other ways to help prevent nausea and vomiting include eating only a light meal before chemotherapy, eating small amounts of food or liquid at a time, eating dry crackers when you feel nauseated, limit liquids with meals but maintain hydration between meals, drink clear liquids like water, apple juice, herbal tea or bouillon, eat cool foods or foods at room temperature, avoid foods with strong odors, avoid foods that are high in fat, fried or greasy, avoid spicy foods, avoid alcohol and caffeine.

The general rule of thumb is that if you cannot keep any foods or liquids down for 12 hours or are only taking in tiny amounts of food or liquids in a 24 hour period, then call your doctor.

16. **DIARRHEA AND CRAMPING**:

For people with pancreatic cancer, diarrhea and cramping can occur for many reasons. They can be caused by a blockage of the bile duct, gallbladder attack, gallstones, pancreatitis, chemotherapy, radiation and medications used to treat the cancer and its symptoms. Diarrhea can cause dehydration, so it is important to talk to your doctor about it in order to take the right antidiarrheal medications at the right time.

Also, eat small amounts of foods or liquids at a time. Increase your fluid intake when having diarrhea and take clear liquids like Gatorade to replace electrolytes. Avoid raw fruits and vegetables, avoid vegetables that cause gas (i.e., beans). Eat bananas, applesauce, canned cooked fruits with the skin removed, white potatoes without the skin, cooked squash or carrots and tomato paste or tomato puree. Avoid alcohol, caffeine and high fiber foods, foods high in lactose (milk, ice cream, cheese). Have lactose free milk, hard cheese, yogurt and sorbet. Avoid fatty, greasy and fried foods and limit butters and oils.

17. **MUCOSITIS OR STOMATITIS**:
Sores and ulcers can occur in the mouth due to chemotherapy. Chemotherapy kills cells that have a fast "turnover" rate. Since chemotherapy cannot target only cancer cells, all cells in the body that have a higher turnover rate are affected. This includes the cells in the mouth. It may be possible to lower the chemotherapy dose if the ulcers and sores become intolerable.

Other ways to prevent ulcers or sores in the mouth include using a soft bristled toothbrush, keeping the mouth moist, rinsing your mouth regularly with a warm saltwater solution, avoiding commercial mouthwashes, avoiding alcohol, eating soft foods, drinking liquid nutritional supplements if swallowing foods becomes intolerable, avoiding hot foods and hot liquids, avoiding foods that irritate the membranes like alcohol, citrus, tomatoes, spices and rough course foods.

If swallowing medication is difficult, ask your doctor for liquid versions of your medication or if you can crush any of your particular medications and mix the crushed medicine with liquid or applesauce.

18. **ANEMIA**:

Chemotherapy treatment for pancreatic cancer can lower your red blood cell count. If the red blood cell count drops too low, you may experience fatigue, shortness of breath, pallor and lightheadedness. Ask your doctor if you can take iron and vitamin supplements. Red blood cell count may be able to be boosted by a prescription of Epogen or Procrit, but those medications also will increase blood pressure, blood clots and mortality.

19. **LOW PLATELET COUNT**:

Chemotherapy treatment for pancreatic cancer can lower your blood platelet count which increases the risk of bleeding. If you are receiving chemotherapy, ask your doctor about avoiding products with aspirin or avoiding NSAIDS like Ibuprofen. If your platelet count drops very low, you may be told to use only an electric razor and avoid activities in which you could be injured. It is important to contact your doctor if you develop signs of excessive bleeding like bruising easily, having bleeding gums, experience nose bleeds, have blood in urine or stool or pass black colored stools.

22. **HAND-FOOT SYNDROME**:

Chemotherapy can cause Hand-Foot Syndrome which can cause tenderness, dryness, redness, and peeling of the palms of the hands and soles of the feet. The skin in these areas consist of cells that have a high turnover rate. Since chemotherapy targets cells with a higher turnover rate, the hands and feet can be affected by chemotherapy. To minimize these symptoms, use a moisturizer and ask your doctor about using ice packs on these surfaces. Also, wear cotton socks and gloves and avoid injuring these areas.

23. **CHEMOTHERAPY-INDUCED PERIPHERAL NEUROPATHY (CIPN)**:

Chemotherapy can damage nerves that are located farther away from the brain and spinal cord (peripheral nerves). These nerves are responsible for controlling the arms, legs, bladder and bowel.

Symptoms of CIPN can include pain, burning, tingling, loss of feeling, trouble grasping, trouble balancing, trouble walking, having a higher sensitivity to heat, cold, touch or pressure, muscle wasting and weakness, trouble swallowing, constipation, trouble urinating, blood pressure changes and reflex changes. If it gets really bad, it can change your heart rate, give you trouble breathing, cause paralysis or even cause organ failure. Contact your doctor if you notice symptoms and the chemotherapy treatment may need to be adjusted.

Generally, the symptoms will first occur in places farthest from the head (i.e., feet first and/or hands first) and then progress up the legs or arms closer toward the head over time. As soon as you notice any symptoms, let your doctor know. Usually, most symptoms will resolve after chemotherapy is discontinued, but some symptoms may become permanent.

Your doctor may adjust your chemotherapy treatment or keep a watch over your CIPN symptoms depending on what type of symptoms you have. The doctor may prescribe steroids, pain medications and anti-seizure medications to address the nerve issues. The doctor may prescribe other types of treatment to assist with CIPN like electrical nerve stimulation, physical therapy, etc…

24. **COGNITIVE ISSUES:**

Pancreatic cancer, treatment for pancreatic cancer and end of life issues due to pancreatic cancer can bring cognitive changes. Depending on the person and how they respond to the cancer, treatment and end of life - some of these cognitive changes can be permanent, but for most people they are temporary.

Chemo Brain:

"Chemo Brain" is what patients experience during chemotherapy treatment. The chemotherapy drugs can cause a generalized haziness in thinking. Some people may experience forgetfulness, trouble recalling some things, an inability to concentrate, inability to multitask or have trouble finding the right words when ending sentences.

Cancer Treatment - Cognitive Issues:

Medications other than chemotherapy used to treat pancreatic cancer may also cause cognitive changes similar to "Chemo Brain".

Pancreatic Cancer - Cognitive Issues:

Pancreatic cancer itself changes the metabolism and can also result in physical changes which alter how the body digests and absorbs nutrients. These physical changes have the ability to cause some cognitive issues with some patients which can be best described as a "foggy brain".

End of Life Cognitive Issues:

When cancer patients are close to death, they often will experience metabolic changes that alter their cognitive state. Patients may become confused or not recognize their friends and family. If this occurs, it is important to announce your name each time you speak to the patient to gently remind them of who you are (but do not argue with them). At the end of my father's life, he at one point thought my brother was someone else and also had asked me a few times where he was (he was in the hospital).

Many will experience hallucinations or talk to people who are not there (or who have predeceased them). During his last full day of being awake, my father thought I had planned a party in the hospital for the American Legion so that his friends could come see him, he saw flying turkeys out the window and he wanted to know what the white stuff was in the tree tops outside of his window. Since he was in such a happy mood, I did not try to tell him that he was wrong or incorrect. I went along with his hallucinations. At the time, my thinking was that he was happy and did not have much time left, and he was enjoying what he was experiencing - so why ruin it for him. After some research, it appears that it is better to go along with the good hallucinations and to call a doctor or nurse if the patient starts having hallucinations that cause them worry or distress.

As death approaches, most patients will become less and less responsive until they eventually drift off into a coma as their body prepares to die.

25. **HAIR THINNING OR HAIR LOSS**:

Chemotherapy has a greater effect on cells that rapidly divide like cells that are responsible for producing hair. When these cells die due to chemotherapy, hair thinning or hair loss can occur. Once the chemotherapy treatment is stopped, hair usually will grow back. Having hair is important to most people as it is a subconscious indicator of health and vitality. In other words, elderly people are generally the ones who tend to have thinning hair or are bald. If hair loss is a concern, then wear hats, wigs or both until your hair has grown back.

26. **FLU-LIKE SYMPTOMS**:

A common side effect of chemotherapy is having flu-like symptoms of muscle pain, fever, headache, chills and fatigue. Since it can be difficult to differentiate between this side effect and actual infection, it is important to notify your doctor if you have any of these symptoms and let your doctor take blood tests to determine what is occurring.

27. **SKIN AND NAIL CHANGES**:

Chemotherapy may produce the following changes to your skin or nails: rash, dry skin, flush skin (temporary redness of the face and neck), hyperpigmentation (darkening of skin), skin itchiness, discoloration of or banding of the nails or nail malformations. Notify your doctor about any changes.

Keep your body hydrated, skin hydrated and keep your skin protected from sun exposure and extreme weather conditions. Keep your hands clean and try to wear as much cotton clothing as possible. Take showers or short cooler baths instead of long hot baths. Do not shave areas of affected skin.

On a daily basis, many of us use perfumed hand soap, dish soap, clothing detergent, moisturizer, shampoo and conditioner, shaving cream, perfume, body spray, deodorant, feminine products, etc... While you have pancreatic cancer or are receiving chemotherapy, it is helpful to avoid perfumed products or other harsh products. It is possible for your skin to become more sensitive to products or detergents that your skin was not sensitive to pre-chemo or pre-cancer. Take inventory of all of your perfumed products and try to switch to less toxic and unscented products.

28. **DIABETES, FRANK DIABETES (HIGH BLOOD SUGAR)**:

The pancreas is responsible for producing insulin which affects affect blood sugar levels. A tumor can impair the pancreas' ability to produce insulin and cause higher blood sugar levels in pancreatic cancer patients. If the Pancreas is surgically removed or partially removed, that can also affect blood sugar levels. Treatments for pancreatic cancer can also affect blood sugar levels. It will be important for your doctor to monitor your blood sugar levels and provide you with insulin medication should you need it. If the entire Pancreas is removed, then diabetes will result and the patient will need monitoring and medication for the rest of their lives. If pancreatic cancer or treatment causes blood sugar levels to drop, then patients may need sugar pills to increase sugar if it gets low while at home.

CHAPTER THIRTEEN

SURGICAL PROCEDURES THAT MAY BE NEEDED FOR THOSE WITH PANCREATIC CANCER

Surgical interventions are used for patients who have pancreatic cancer; however, only if they meet certain qualifications. Doctors try to balance the severity of the particular issue (i.e., degree of intestinal blockage), the stage of cancer, the age of the patient, the overall prognosis of the cancer, the presence of ascites and the patient's performance status. The patient's wishes are also considered.

There appear to be two main stages in the progression of pancreatic cancer. The "first stage" is where a patient with pancreatic cancer is still strong, has months to live and can withstand surgical intervention. The "second stage" is where a patient's health has greatly deteriorated, the patient is in the end stage of the cancer with probably only weeks to live, and the patient would probably not tolerate surgical intervention. Usually, patients voluntarily forego surgical intervention when they are in the "second stage" because they want to spend what time they have left in a state of comfort with their family and friends without hastening their death with chemotherapy or surgery.

1. **STENTS FOR BILE DUCT BLOCKAGE AND INTESTINAL BLOCKAGE**:

Bile Duct Blockage:
A stent is a short tube (it can be a tube with holes or a solid tube). Stents are inserted into areas of the body in order to maintain the flow of biological "traffic". For example, a stent may be placed in a blocked artery in order to unblock it and maintain a good flow of blood to the heart.

Many pancreatic cancer patients will end up having a blockage in their bile duct because the tumor in the head of the pancreas may squeeze the bile duct shut (or may even invade the bile duct). Stents are preferred to bile duct bypass because they are less invasive; however, each stent procedure can have a cumulative effect on weakening the body.

Those who have pancreatic cancer should not have any metal stents placed in their bile duct until they have been completely evaluated for Whipple surgery. Once a metal stent is put into the bile duct it cannot be removed and it makes having the Whipple surgery almost impossible. Metal stents are generally used when surgery is not an option because they tend to last longer than plastic stents. Plastic stents are usually used when Whipple Surgery may be a future possibility.

Stents are prone to occlusion (being blocked) and plastic stents usually need to be replaced at 3 month intervals. Metal stents also usually become occluded after about 8-12 months and are usually used on those who do not qualify for the Whipple surgery and whose life expectancy is not anticipated to be very long. If necessary, it may be possible to unblock an occluded metal stent.

The types of conditions that can block a stent include: gallstone, gallbladder sludge, microbial biofilm growth, infection, tumor growth into the stent, tumor growth at either end of the stent, and duodenal (small intestines) reflux of food into the bile duct and stent.

A complication of having stents is cholangitis, an infection of the bile duct. This complication can further weaken the body and the infection may travel into the liver and/or cause death.

Before you have an ERCP procedure to remove a gallstone or to treat a blocked bile duct due to pancreatic cancer - ask the doctors what type of stent they intend to use. Make sure they are using a plastic stent if you have not been evaluated for the Whipple procedure. If they intend to use a metal stent, find out what type it is as "covered" metal stents can aid in removal or repositioning and self-expanding metal stents (SEMS) may help prevent occlusion. Talk to your doctor about your medical condition, what types of stents are available and what stents would be most appropriate (and why).

My father had what they thought was a gallstone blocking his bile duct (he had painless jaundice). They attempted an ERCP procedure to remove the stone and they couldn't remove it. They thought the stone was impacted in his bile duct. They sent him to an expert for another ERCP and that expert removed the stone and put a metal stent in my father's bile duct. I do not know if anyone ever gave my father notice that they might stent him. I don't think he was given an option on what type of stent would be placed inside of him.

One of his doctors eventually told me that he had a metal stent inside of him. I do not know if it was a covered metal stent, an expanding metal stent or just a plain metal stent. My father's stent appeared to have become occluded within a few weeks' time. I do not know if it was occluded by a gallstone, by infection, by sludge, by the tumor putting pressure on a different part of the bile duct or by an inflamed pancreas putting pressure on part of the bile duct (due to acute pancreatitis).

An example of a metal stent would be the Boston Scientific Wallstent. Under product warnings, it states that complications from using it in the bile duct include "infection, stent misplacement, stent migration, stent obstruction secondary to tumor in-growth through the stent, tumor overgrowth at the stent ends or sludge occlusion."

Another example of a metal stent is the Gore Viabil Stent. It lists its long term patency rates at 96% at 3 months, 85% at 6 months and 72% as 12 months. This means that at 12 months, 72% of the stents were not occluded and still operating well inside of the bile duct.

Pancreatic Duct Blockage:

Stents are not usually placed in a narrowed or blocked pancreatic duct because the stents tend to migrate, penetrate the pancreas, cause pancreatitis and also need to be replaced very often.

Intestinal Blockage:

As discussed in the last chapter, pancreatic cancer tumors can cause a blockage of the intestines by growing into the intestines or pressing down and squeezing the intestines shut. The preferred method of resolving an intestinal blockage if medications do not work is using self-expanding metallic stents (SEMS) to open the blockage.

If stenting does not work, then an intestinal resection may have to be performed. With an intestinal resection, the surgeon will open up the abdomen, try to clear the blockage, and if he cannot clear it he may need to cut the blockage out and reconnect the ends of two healthy sections of intestines together. It is possible that if the intestines have "died" and cannot be reconnected that the doctor will need to form a "stoma" to drain the intestinal contents into a bag on the outside of the body.

With pancreatic cancer, the surgeon may need to remove part of the intestine or part of the pancreatic tumor or both in order to resolve the bowel obstruction.

2. **SURGICAL BYPASS**:

    Bile Duct Blockage:
    If the bile duct becomes blocked because the tumor is pressing on it and a stent fails, surgeons may perform a bile duct bypass. With a bile duct bypass, a surgeon will cut the bile duct tube and redirect the flow of bile elsewhere in the body or even into a bag hanging outside of the body. The purpose is to relieve jaundice and/or cholangitis (an infection in the bile duct).

    Intestinal Obstruction:
    If the tumor grows into the small intestines (duodenum) and blocks the passage of food, surgeons can perform a bypass to relieve the blockage.

3. **NERVE BLOCK**:
    If significant pain develops because the pancreatic cancer tumor is invading the nerve bundle known as the Celiac Plexus, then doctors usually can easily perform a nerve block where alcohol is injected into the nerve bundle to relieve the pain. Having this minor surgery can help reduce the need for opiods.

4. **PARTIAL REMOVAL OF PANCREATIC TUMOR**:
    If possible, surgeons will remove the tumor in what is called the Whipple surgery. If the pancreatic duct is blocked, then the patient may suffer from chronic pancreatitis due to pancreatic enzymes backing up inside of the

pancreas, activating and then digesting the pancreas itself. To prevent further pancreatitis attacks, part of the pancreas may be removed.

5. **ASCITES**:

   For some pancreatic cancer patients, ascites will begin to occur during the end stages of the cancer. Ascites is simply the buildup of fluid in the abdomen. This buildup of fluid can cause various discomforts to the patient. To temporarily relieve the discomfort, doctors have traditionally prescribed diuretics or drained the fluid (Paracentesis). Draining the fluid is usually only a temporary measure and cannot be done too often because it saps the body of energy and proteins. More current treatments include implanting a pleurx catheter to help drain the fluid if the ascites is recurring rapidly and is interfering with breathing.

6. **GALBLADDER REMOVAL:**

   The gallbladder will be removed if it becomes inflamed or if gallstones threaten to block the bile duct.

CHAPTER FOURTEEN

SCREENINGS AND ONGOING SCREENINGS:

Pancreatic cancer patients should speak with their treating physicians about ongoing screenings in order to determine if current treatments are working and to determine future treatment options. The time intervals for the screenings vary and are based on the patient's specific needs.

1. **Metastasis Screenings**: PET and CT Scan with Contrast and Ultrasound can be used to determine if the cancer has metastasized to other parts of the body.

2. **Bowel Obstruction Screenings**: This screening should be performed if there is a risk that the bowel could become obstructed due to symptoms, where the tumor is located, projected tumor growth and medical treatments that have been used.

3. **Stent Failure Screenings**: This screening should be performed if a stent is placed within the gastrointestinal tract. Stent failure screenings would include testing to see if any occlusion of the stent or stent migration is occurring.

4. **Pancreas Fluids Screening**: This screening should be performed depending on where the tumor is growing and its growth rate. If the pancreatic duct has shown narrowing or is predicted to narrow, then this screening should be used to determine whether or not supplemental pancreatic enzymes should be taken and whether the patient should start to eat very small meals more frequently as opposed to larger meals three times a day.

5. **Blood - CBC and Liver Panel Screenings**: These screenings and provide results as to overall health and give clues as to what is occurring internally.

6. **Cancer CA19-9 Marker Screening**: CA19-9 is a protein that is found in the blood of some pancreatic cancer patients. This screening is effective for

SOME people AFTER they have been diagnosed with pancreatic cancer. Not everyone is sensitive to this biomarker. For those who are, measuring the CA19-9 marker in the blood can help determine if treatments are working to eradicate the cancer. If a treatment is working, the CA19-9 level tends to go down.

7. **Tumor Growth or Receding Screening**: This screening can help determine if surgery is a possibility. For some patients, chemotherapy can help shrink a pancreatic cancer tumor to the point where surgery may be possible. This screening can also determine the course of treatment for the prevention of a bile duct blockage.

8. **Diabetes and Blood Sugar Screenings**: This screening can help determine whether the tumor is interfering with the pancreas' ability to produce insulin.

9. **Screening for other cancers** as other cancers can be associated with pancreatic cancer. This can affect treatment options.

10. **Ascites Screening**: This screening can help determine whether ascites exists and if further anti-cancer treatment should be continued. This screening can also assist with preventing breathing problems associated with some cases of ascites.

11. **Blood Clots**: This screening can help determine whether blood thinning medications should be taken or continued.

12. **Infections - Pancreas, Gallbladder, Liver, Bile Duct (Cholangitis)**: It is very important that pancreatic cancer patients communicate with their doctors about any signs of infection so that the infection can be treated right away.

CHAPTER FIFTEEN

WHEN SHOULD AN ER VISIT BE MADE

At the start of my father's cancer journey, I wish I had made a chart for when I should have called an ambulance or his doctor. The problem was, at times I was not sure whether or not I should call an ambulance. Of course, always err on the side of caution – but it would have been nice to have a chart outlining when an ambulance or doctor should be contacted. In addition to the normal reasons to call an ambulance (chest pain, shortness of breath, passing out, numbness in limbs, etc...) – discuss with your doctor when an ambulance should be called. Here are some factors you may want to discuss with him.

1. **Intolerable Pain**

2. **Leg Swelling**: Could be caused by DVT so if it happens in one leg with redness, heat or pain then go to ER.

3. **Significant Unusual Bleeding**:
   Easy bruising, bleeding gums, nose bleeds, blood in urine or stool and if you have black stools.

4. **Blood Pressure Readings**:   Too low _____ or too high _____
   (according to limits set by your doctor)

5. **Blood Sugar Readings**:   Too low _____ or too high _____
   (according to limits set by your doctor)

6. **Vomiting**:   Vomiting continuously for _____ long

7. **Nausea**:   Nauseous for _____ long

8. **Diarrhea**:   Continuous for _____ days

8. **Urine Color**:   Dark Colored?   Unable to urinate

9. **Stool Color**: Clay Colored? Black Colored? Bloody? Unable to Defecate for _____ Hours/Days?

10. **Fever**: Above _____ degrees

11. **Chills and/or Night Sweats**

12. **Unusual Itching**

13. **Feeling Faint/Passing Out**

14. **Food Consumption**: Unable to eat for _____ hours

15. **Fluids**: Unable to drink for _____ hours

16. **Weight Loss**: Weight Loss of more than _____ pounds.

CHAPTER SIXTEEN

SUPPORT

Pancreatic cancer patients need SUPPORT. The following list should be filled out with important names and phone numbers that can fulfill various needs that the patient may have throughout his illness. Look up various resources in your area on the internet. Also talk to each contact about further resources they may be aware of that can help.

1. **Doctors / Treatment Team**:
   Primary Care Physician Name/Address/Phone:
   Medical Oncologist Name/Address/Phone:
   Surgical Oncologist Name/Address/Phone:
   Palliative Care Physician Name/Address/Phone:
   Local Hospital Name/Address/Phone:
   Pharmacy Name/Address/Phone:
   Emergency Numbers:

2. **Family and Friends**

3. **Support Groups and/or Therapist**

4. **Hospices**

5. **Non Emergency 24 Hour Support Line for Info (See Health Insurance Company Phone Contact)**:

6. **Support Help/Referrals**:

    1. Senior Services:

    2. Caregiving Volunteers:

    4. County Services:

    5. American Cancer Society: counseling, equipment, supplies, transportation assistance, financial aid for medications

    6. Hospital:

    7. Board of Social Services:

    8. Home Health Care Agencies:

7. **Medical Supplies**:

    1. Hospice:

    2. Caregiving Volunteers:

    3. Elks:

8. **Nutritional**:

    Nutritional Management Doctor/Nurse:

9. **Transportation:**

    1. American Cancer Society:

    2. Hospital:

    3. County Board of Social Services:

10. **Social Worker**:

    1. Groceries:

    2. Transportation to Appointments:

11. **At Home Nurse Care**:

12. **Home Health Aid**:

CHAPTER SEVENTEEN

HOSPICE AND THE DYING PROCESS

Most people diagnosed with pancreatic cancer will succumb to the disease. At a point in time, it will be pointless to continue fruitless treatments that negatively affect the quality of life the person has left. At this time, doctors will recommend that patients seek hospice care.

Hospice care is end of life care. The patient gives up all life-saving cancer treatment (i.e., chemotherapy) and 100% of the care provided is focused on keeping the person as comfortable as possible until they pass. For my father, this meant lots of morphine. For others, it may mean that they get their regular blood pressure medication, treatment for ascites, a pain patch and the addition of morphine at the end stages of the disease.

It helps to research different hospices in your area ahead of time. Most people prefer to have hospice in their homes so they can be comfortable. Hospice will normally provide a hospital bed, nurses who will visit for a short period every day and medication that is needed for comfort. Some hospices are located in their own building or as part of a hospital. Generally speaking, most health insurance will cover hospice care 100%.

My dad was only on hospice for about 3 days before he died. Some people can be on hospice for 6 months or more.

In the hospital, when my father was told that there was really no more they could do for him, they recommended hospice at home. My father was in a weakened state and frightened. He never really had the time to even digest that he had pancreatic cancer. When I asked him if he would like me to take him home on hospice, he said, "No, I want to stay here (the hospital). If I go home I will be in pain and miserable." I reassured him that he wouldn't be in pain and miserable, but that he didn't have to even be concerned about it at that point because he had time to decide whatever it is he wanted to do.

I contacted the hospice nurse and asked her to meet with him a couple of days later to explain to him what hospice was and what it would do for him so that he didn't have fears about it. A couple of days later he was completely unconscious and never was able to meet with the hospice nurse. I signed him into hospice care; however, all of his hospice care occurred in the hospital because it took the hospital days to have his pain completely managed.

The point of researching hospice ahead of time is so that the person who has pancreatic cancer can feel more comfortable knowing all of his or her options - and have more control over the entire process.

The Dying Process

A doctor cannot tell you when someone will die. They can provide an estimate, but the estimate is often wrong. To avoid angering patients and families, doctors will often avoid answering the question "How much time is left before he dies?"

Although everyone dies in varying ways, there are some "norms" for people who die from cancer. The following information applies only those who are "pre-actively" or "actively" dying (usually the last couple of weeks of life).

There are all sorts of variables within the "norm", but generally speaking:

1. **Pre-Active Phase of Dying**:
   In the pre-active phase of dying, people will spend a number of weeks sleeping in or napping more often. They won't eat or drink as much as they normally do.

2. **Appetite and Thirst**:
   The first thing to start to "go" when someone is actively dying is appetite and thirst. You will notice that the person's appetite starts to decrease and eventually it will get to a point where they have no desire to eat or drink. The rule of thumb is to ALWAYS allow the actively dying cancer patient to decide when to eat, what to eat and how much to eat (or drink). NEVER force food or drink on them. When the body is preparing to die, it purposely prevents the cancer patient from being hungry or thirsty so that the gastrointestinal system can start to shut down. By forcing food, you can

make this shutting down process a lot more painful and uncomfortable for the actively dying cancer patient. My dad, along with most patients, prefer just having a small ice chip placed in the mouth to keep it feeling moist and comfortable. You won't want to place anything in anyone's mouth other than a sponge with a bit of moisture on it once the actively dying person is unconscious - otherwise you can cause aspiration, choking, etc...

3. **Consciousness**:

It takes a lot of energy to be "awake", "see" and "converse" with others. After the appetite and thirst disappear, then the person will fall asleep and cannot be wakened from that sleep. The patient will be in a coma-like state. It is presumed throughout the entire dying process that hearing is the last sense to go - so it is important not to say upsetting things within earshot of the dying person. It's even better if you can "pretend" the dying person is present and able to hear regardless of his apparent state of consciousness. Never talk about the dying person while he is laying there. Talk to him as though he is there and conscious.

At this time COMFORT is KEY. Play music, turn on the television to his favorite channel, talk to him, hold his hand and lightly rub areas where he should not experience pain (for my dad, we avoided his belly area and lightly rubbed his shoulder, his head or his hand). Keep his mouth moist - remoisten it at least once an hour (the nurses can show you how). Make sure his body is comfortable. If you notice shivering, get him blankets. If he's sweating or overly hot - remove blankets. If his arm is swelling, remove constricted objects. Remove his eyeglasses. Make sure his body is in a comfortable position in the bed (with a supported head, back and neck).

The nurses can show you other ways to make him comfortable. One of the most important things is to watch for signs of cringing in his face or stiffening up of his arms or body movements. If any of these events happen, immediately notify a nurse that he needs more pain medication right away. During this time, he can experience pain and comfort, but he will NOT be able to communicate verbally with you. It is vital that he is paid attention to for signals of pain or discomfort and that that any indications of pain or discomfort be attended to right away.

4. **Swelling**:

After the loss of consciousness, the next thing you may notice is swelling in the limbs and/or face. As the circulatory system slows down and the kidneys start to shut themselves down - body fluids become imbalanced and swelling can occur. I would recommend that all jewelry and watches should be removed once someone becomes unconscious because swelling happens quite often and can happen overnight. This swelling is a normal part of the dying process, but comfort measures should be taken. Swollen limbs should be slightly elevated, restricted clothing items or jewelry should be removed, the swollen parts of the body should not be touched or rubbed because the swelling can cause a problem with skin integrity - rubbing or touching the swollen skin could cause pain or other problems for your loved one.

5. **Open Mouth Breathing**:

   The next part of actively dying usually involves the person breathing through their mouth. Eventually, the person will start to breath with the mouth wide open along with mandibular (jaw) movement. This means that the person will become slack jawed as their muscles completely relax. The jaw/chin will move a little with each breath.

5. **Breathing Rate Changes**:

   Breathing rate changes will eventually start to occur. Cheyne-Stokes Breathing is when deeper breaths are taken and the breathing pattern will sometimes speed up or slow down. A sleep apnea may occur where the breathing will stop for a few seconds or more and then resume.

   The "death rattle" may occur. This is simply a gurgling sound that originates in the throat. It can be difficult to listen to, but it causes no discomfort to the patient. The death rattle is common, but may not occur if the patient has been given medication to reduce fluids being produced in his mouth and throat.

   At the end of life, my father's breathing was pretty stable right until the last few minutes of death. During the last few minutes of death, each breath was extremely shallow with a long pause in between his breaths.

6. **Cooler Limbs**:

    As the body shuts down, the circulation shuts down as well. As some people approach death, their limbs will become cooler to the touch.

7. **Fever**:

    As the body shuts down, the temperature regulating region of the brain may go haywire and the dying person may experience fevers. Medication to reduce fever (via suppositories) may be provided to give comfort.

8. **Urine and Bowel Movement Changes**:

    As the body shuts down, the dying person may have a reduction in urine output and bowel movements. In addition, the urine that is expelled may become darker.

9. **Mottling of the Skin**:

    An imminent sign of death is the mottling of certain areas of the skin. The mottling is a purplish blotchiness that occurs on the parts of the body as a result of blood pooling (lack of circulation). Near the time of death, most people are lying on their backs and so the mottling can occur on the heels of the feet and along their entire backside in places. On the morning of his death, my father had mottling on the heels of his feet. He didn't pass away until about 6 pm that evening.

CHAPTER TWENTY

LEGAL DOCUMENTS

When it was time for my dad to be put into hospice, it was the hardest thing that I ever had to do in my life. I felt like I was responsible for his death, although I knew it was for the best. He was unconscious at that time and was never to regain consciousness again. Thankfully, he had given me what's called a **"Health Care Power of Attorney"** which gave me the ability to sign his hospice paperwork since he was unable to. This document prevented family fights and enabled my father to have a smooth transition into hospice care. The document can also be used to limit visitors and to access medical records to make informed medical decisions for your loved one.

I also was able to use a "Durable Power of Attorney" that my dad had prepared which allowed me to withdraw money from his savings account to pay a deposit for the funeral. A Durable Power of Attorney expires as soon as a person dies. Once a person dies, the Executor/Executrix named in the deceased's Last Will and Testament has the powers over the estate. Again, I was named the Executrix in my dad's Will and was able to file for Probate and have myself named as Executrix of his estate so that I could wrap up his estate.

For the legal paperwork, every state's requirements are different. The following forms are for general guidelines only. Hiring an expensive attorney isn't necessary if you do the research and ensure your documents conform to whatever your state laws require. It's also important to choose people you absolutely trust to carry out your wishes.

The Recommended End of Life Documents:

1. **Last Will and Testament**

    A will becomes effective upon your death. This document lets everyone know your wishes and makes it easier for your family to settle your estate after death.

2. **Durable Power of Attorney**

    A Durable Power of Attorney can become effective at any time – and in my dad's case, his document was written to become effective once he could no longer make decisions for himself.

    This document allows you to appoint someone to take care of all of your affairs if for some reason you cannot do it yourself. This includes accessing all of your financial accounts and even possibly selling your home (if the monies are needed for long term care). A Durable Power of Attorney becomes effective when someone is incapable of taking care of things himself (i.e., bed bound, unconscious or medically incompetent).

3. **Health Care Power of Attorney**

   This document allows you to appoint someone to make health care decisions for you if you are unable to do so (i.e., unconscious or mentally incompetent). This document can be used to hospitalize you, transfer you to hospice, get you treatment, limit visitors, transfer you to a nursing home, and to obtain access to your medical records to make competent decisions on your behalf and in accordance with your wishes.

4. **Funeral Representative**

   This document allows you to appoint someone to make decisions on how your body will be taken care of once you are deceased. The person can decide if you are to have a viewing, a funeral, be buried or cremated.

5. **Living Will**

   This document communicates your wishes for your healthcare to your doctors and your family. Most elderly people choose to have a "do not resuscitate" order on their medical chart because medical resuscitation can be very brutal and is often fruitless at end of life. You may wish to have all necessary measures taken to keep you alive (i.e., feeding tube, ventilation) or choose to forego a feeding tube and ventilation when end of life is apparent. Give a copy of this to your local hospital and doctor once it is signed. All of your documents should be kept in a safe place that can be accessible by the person(s) you trust to provide end of life care.

Please note that the HIPPA form which the pancreatic cancer patient may sign designating others to have access to his or her records ONLY gives access to medical records. It does NOT give anyone the right to make medical decisions on his behalf.

I wrote this book for other pancreatic cancer patients and their loved ones. I wanted to provide a resource to help them navigate the labyrinth of pancreatic cancer. After extensive research, I am very optimistic that in 10 years, we will be able to vastly expand the lives of those with pancreatic cancer. The scientific efforts on research and development in this disease is skyrocketing. The deaths of famous people are also bringing pancreatic cancer to the forefront. These people include Patrick Swayze, Steve Jobs and more recently I believe David Bowie died from it as well.

Pancreatic cancer is highly deadly. It seems silly to tell pancreatic cancer patients not to give up hope because in many cases (like my father's) it was hopeless. I think it would be more appropriate to remind pancreatic patients that if you qualify for treatment, then it is possible to live longer than 3-6 months. There are people with pancreatic cancer who have reached the 3 year mark of life, the 5 year mark and beyond.

Printed in Great Britain
by Amazon